Mastering Forensic Psychiatric Practice

Advanced Strategies for the Expert Witness

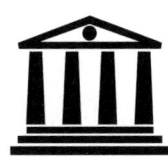

Mastering Forensic Psychiatric Practice

Advanced Strategies for the Expert Witness

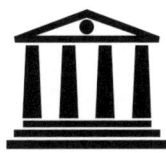

Thomas G. Gutheil, M.D.
Robert I. Simon, M.D.

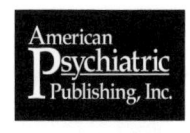

Washington, DC
London, England

Note: The authors have worked to ensure that all information in this book concerning drug dosages, schedules, and routes of administration is accurate as of the time of publication and consistent with standards set by the U.S. Food and Drug Administration and the general medical community. As medical research and practice advance, however, therapeutic standards may change. For this reason and because human and mechanical errors sometimes occur, we recommend that readers follow the advice of a physician who is directly involved in their care or the care of a member of their family. A product's current package insert should be consulted for full prescribing and safety information.

Books published by American Psychiatric Publishing, Inc., represent the views and opinions of the individual authors and do not necessarily represent the policies and opinions of APPI or the American Psychiatric Association.

Copyright © 2002 American Psychiatric Publishing, Inc.
ALL RIGHTS RESERVED

Manufactured in Canada on acid-free paper
06 05 04 03 02   5 4 3 2 1
First Edition

American Psychiatric Publishing, Inc.
1400 K Street, N.W.
Washington, DC 20005
www.appi.org

Library of Congress Cataloging-in-Publication Data
Gutheil, Thomas G.
  Mastering forensic psychiatric practice : advanced strategies for the expert witness / Thomas G. Gutheil, Robert I. Simon.—1st ed.
    p. ; cm.
  Includes bibliographical references and index.
  ISBN 1-58562-007-6 (alk. paper)
  1. Forensic psychiatry. 2. Evidence, Expert. I. Simon, Robert I. II. Title.
  [DNLM: 1. Forensic Psychiatry—United States. 2. Expert Testimony—methods—United States. W740 G984m 2002]
  RA1151 .G884 2002
  614'.1—dc21

2001056176

British Library Cataloguing in Publication Data
A CIP record is available from the British Library.

*To our students and colleagues,
who have taught us so much*

Contents

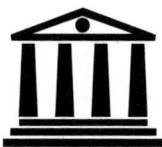

About the Authors xi

Preface....................................... xiii

Acknowledgments xvii

PART I
Introduction and Basics

1 The Expert's Task 3

PART II
Practical Matters

2 Practical Aspects of the Forensic Examination 13

Appendix 2–1: A Model Consent Form 21

3 Boundary Issues in Case Preparation
With Attorneys................................. 23

4 Fee Agreements and Finances in Forensic Practice:
Theoretical and Empirical Dimensions.............. 31

Appendix 4–1: Model Fee Agreement Guidelines 41

PART III
Problem Areas in Attorney-Expert Relations

5 Attorneys' Pressures on the Expert Witness: Early Warning Signs and Empirical Study of Endangered Honesty and Objectivity 47

6 The Phantom Expert: Use of an Expert's Name or Alleged Testimony Without Consent as a Legal Strategy. 67

PART IV
Forensic Countertransference

7 Issues in Forensic Countertransference: Early Warning Signs of Compromised Distance and Objectivity. 81

PART V
Problems With Deposition and Trial Testimony

8 Personal Questions on Cross-Examination: A Pilot Study of Expert Witness Attitudes 93

9 Telling Tales Out of Court: Experts' Disclosures About Opposing Experts 101

10 Effects of the *Daubert* Case on Preparing Psychiatric/Psychological Testimony for Court 113

PART VI
Ethical Issues

11 Some Ethical Dilemmas 127

Appendix 11–1: American Academy of Psychiatry and the Law Ethical Guidelines for the Practice of Forensic Psychiatry 135

Epilogue. 141

Suggested Readings 143

Index 145

About the Authors

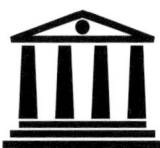

Thomas G. Gutheil, M.D., is Professor of Psychiatry at Harvard Medical School, Co-Director of the Program in Psychiatry and the Law at the Massachusetts Mental Health Center, Past President of the American Academy of Psychiatry and the Law, and a Fellow of the American Psychiatric Association. He is the first Professor of Psychiatry in the history of Harvard Medical School to be board certified in both general and forensic psychiatry. Through more than 200 publications and international lectures and seminars, he has taught many clinicians about the interfaces between psychiatry and the law. Recipient of every major award in the forensic field, he has also received local and national teaching awards, and his textbook *Clinical Handbook of Psychiatry and the Law*, coauthored with Paul S. Appelbaum, M.D., received the Manfred S. Guttmacher Award as the outstanding contribution to forensic psychiatric literature.

Robert I. Simon, M.D., is Clinical Professor of Psychiatry and Director, Program in Psychiatry and Law, at Georgetown University School of Medicine in Washington, D.C. Dr. Simon is a Life Fellow of the American Psychiatric Association and board certified in both general and forensic psychiatry. He has received the Manfred S. Guttmacher Award for his outstanding contribution to forensic psychiatry. He has also received the Seymour Pollack Distinguished Achievement Award for distinguished contribution to the field of forensic psychiatry. Dr. Simon has published numerous articles and chapters as well as authored, coauthored, and edited 22 books and editions in forensic psychiatry.

Preface

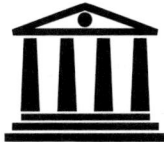

The passage of time has not slowed the growth of interest in forensic work by mental health professionals; rather, this interest has increased. Various factors account for this trend, including the desire for freedom from the constraints of managed care, the intellectual challenge in reconciling the disciplines of psychiatry and law, the possibility of additional income, and the inception of formal certification in forensic work in psychology and psychiatry.

Formal training through accredited forensic fellowships is similarly on the rise. At the time of this writing, the American Academy of Psychiatry and the Law, the national forensic psychiatric association, which boasts nearly 2,500 members, lists 32 accredited forensic fellowships nationwide.

In keeping with the growth of this field, textbooks have begun to appear, directed at those entering the field (1, 2) and current practitioners wishing to learn about it in greater depth (3–8). This book belongs to the latter category. Designed as the conceptual successor to *The Psychiatrist as Expert Witness* (1), this text assumes some familiarity with the basic concepts addressed therein but explores the concerns of the more experienced forensic practitioner. We have further chosen to emphasize here the role of the privately retained expert rather than that of the practitioner employed in an institution, and we have emphasized civil contexts more than criminal ones. However, most of the principles described here would apply equally well to criminal work.

Forensic psychiatry in its early days lacked an empirical tradition. The paucity of "alienists" willing to work with the courts and the largely anecdotal material available from individual practitioners produced a mystifying miscellany of idiosyncratic information for scholars interested in defining the forensic field. With the emergence of professional organizations and peer-reviewed journals, empirical study and both descriptive and prospective research in forensic subjects began to flower.

The practical aspects of forensic work, however, have not often been systematically studied. Here is a unique feature of this book. Unlike other texts in the field, this one contains empirical data on actual forensic practice—data previously unavailable. These new findings provide a sound basis for the recommendations we offer.

Although pilot versions of some of these empirical studies (which appear here with permission) have been previously published in professional journals, the materials have been revised and expanded to chapter length and are assembled here for the first time to allow for a comprehensive overview. The purpose of these studies and of the chapters in which they appear is to provide the experienced expert with a deeper understanding of the forensic field and of the relationship between forensic experts and attorneys. We also seek to open exploration into subject areas that—though invariably the subject of casual discussion at professional meetings—have previously lacked systematic investigation.

In the service of fostering and improving dialogue between the clinical and legal professions, this volume is further intended to be read by attorneys who work with experts in forensic mental health fields. If the information herein diminishes the tensions that can arise between experts and retaining attorneys, the work will have fulfilled one of its purposes.

The authors hope that this and similar works will continue to raise the standards of practice in the forensic field.

Thomas G. Gutheil, M.D.
Robert I. Simon, M.D.

References

1. Gutheil TG: The Psychiatrist as Expert Witness. Washington, DC, American Psychiatric Press, 1998
2. Berger S: Establishing a Forensic Practice. New York, WW Norton, 1997
3. Gutheil TG, Appelbaum PS: Clinical Handbook of Psychiatry and the Law, 3rd Edition. Baltimore, MD, Williams & Wilkins, 2000
4. Rosner R (ed): Principles and Practice of Forensic Psychiatry. London, Arnold Publishers, 1992
5. Simon RI (ed): Review of Clinical Psychiatry and the Law, Vol 1. Washington, DC, American Psychiatric Press, 1990

6. Simon RI (ed): Review of Clinical Psychiatry and the Law, Vol 2. Washington, DC, American Psychiatric Press, 1991
7. Simon RI (ed): Review of Clinical Psychiatry and the Law, Vol 3. Washington, DC, American Psychiatric Press, 1992
8. Simon RI (ed): Posttraumatic Stress Disorder in Litigation. Washington, DC, American Psychiatric Press, 1995

Acknowledgments

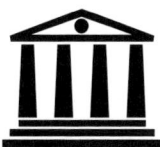

We gratefully acknowledge the support and inspiration of our wives, Shannon Woolley and Patricia Simon; Ellen Lewy's assistance with the manuscript; the participation in the empirical aspects of this book by members of the Program in Psychiatry and the Law at the Massachusetts Mental Health Center, Harvard Medical School, and members of the American Academy of Psychiatry and the Law; the valued contributions of our reviewers; and the unflagging assistance and support of the editorial staff of American Psychiatric Publishing, Inc.

Note on Terminology

In the text, in page citations from direct quotations of legal material, the term *at* preceding page number(s) indicates the exact page(s) on which the quotation is located. In reference lists, in page citations of legal material, the term *at* indicates the page where the reference begins.

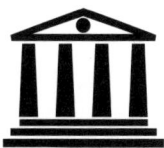

PART I

Introduction and Basics

1

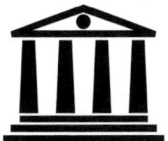

The Expert's Task

> The expert's job at trial is to fill in each color [as in a paint-by-numbers kit] carefully, without concern for the completed painting. The attorney's task is to arrange the colored areas into a meaningful pattern through choices about the order and questioning of witnesses (although before the trial, experts certainly can help the attorney compose parts of the portrait).
>
> M. Mays, in (1), p. 12

The psychiatric expert witness has several roles to play when participating in the legal process. The roles in question may be labeled, in roughly chronological sequence, consultant, businessperson, teacher, advocate, witness, and performer. Below we examine these roles and address the functions peculiar to each.

Consultant

The expert is always functioning as a consultant, but this role is especially clear at the very outset of being retained by the attorney. The expert offers consultation on psychiatry to the attorney, who is not as knowledgeable about that specialty. In fact, the role of consultant must antedate the role of witness, since the expert's review of the relevant materials and consequent opinion will determine whether the attorney can actually use the expert to advance the attorney's side of the case.

A possible point of confusion should be addressed here. Although the expert witness may serve the generic consulting functions described above, the term *consulting witness* (sometimes *nontestifying witness*) may also describe a specific role function that is distinguished from *testifying witness* as follows:

A testifying witness is one who is expected to be available to testify should a case come to trial and whose objective opinion may be obtained through customary discovery mechanisms such as reports, interrogatories, and depositions. A consulting (or nontestifying) expert works behind the scenes, as it were, in a more partisan fashion, advising the attorney in various areas, such as case strategy, weaknesses in the other side, and settlement discussions; the views of the latter type of witness are usually protected from discovery by work-product considerations. Such witnesses probably should not go on to be testifying witnesses because their earlier partisan role may bias their objectivity. But empirical observation attests that some attorneys freely discuss such matters even with testifying witnesses, an action blurring in practice the theoretical distinction just made.

The consultant role of the modern expert witness also includes consultation on opening statement and closing argument. A number of experts function as jury consultants as well, but this role is considered to be in conflict with the role of testifying expert, since, as earlier suggested, one's objectivity may be compromised by assumption of so partisan a role (1, 2).

Businessperson

Except in pro bono work, the expert is entering into a business arrangement with the attorney. This matter should be straightforward—the expert is selling time and consultative services—but can become both pragmatically and emotionally complicated. Some of the vagaries of this business arrangement are discussed in later chapters regarding fee agreements and economic pressures brought to bear on the expert by the attorney.

Teacher

Unquestionably, expert witness practice most closely resembles teaching. The teaching takes place in two well-defined phases.

First, the expert teaches the attorney about the valid psychiatric aspects of the case; about the contributions, if any, that psychiatry can make to the case; about the psychiatric strengths and weaknesses of the attorney's theory of the case; and about what the witness can say regarding these issues to a reasonable degree of medical certainty, the usual expert testimonial standard.

The second phase consists of teaching the jury about the psychiatric issues. This process involves an act of translation, converting psychiatric terms, jargon, and concepts into lay language and imagery; an act of illustration, whereby the expert attempts to make clear, even vivid, the issues at stake; and an act of persuasion, whereby the expert attempts to have the jury see his or her own vision of the matter.

Advocate

The concept of the expert as persuader takes us to the next expert role—that of advocate. There is a delicate distinction to be made here. The expert, having reached an opinion by careful review of the database (totality of case materials, interviews, testimony, etc.) and application of the requisite training and experience, may ethically state his or her *opinion* persuasively. This action must be distinguished from *advocacy for the side of the case that retains the expert,* since that is the attorney's role, not the expert's. The expert has no business advocating for either side of a case. The expert merely testifies under oath to the opinion, regardless of that opinion's frankly admitted limitations and weaknesses; the fact finder decides the outcome.

Indeed, losing perspective on this separate advocacy and consequently becoming invested in the case outcome is a classic occupational hazard for expert witnesses generally. It is hard for the beginning witness to grasp how interest in the outcome of the case constitutes a contaminating bias of the necessary objectivity, but bias it is. The distinction being made is between persuasiveness and advocacy, the former valid, the latter a form of bias.

Witness

Based on a number of factors, only one of which is the expert's opinion, the retaining attorney may decide to declare the expert as a witness; this step commonly involves disclosing the expert's name and credentials in some form and sometimes forecasting what the expert may say at trial. The expert is now directly associated with the case and may expect to participate by means of interrogatories, depositions, and/or trial testimony.

Performer

If the litigation arrives at the stage of actual trial testimony (most cases do not), the expert will play a role that captures the theatrical dimension of courtroom activity (3). Expert witness testimony—especially before a jury but sometimes even before a judge—can, like good teaching, be likened to a kind of performance. Elements of drama and narrative, and evocation of emotions as well as thoughts, are commonly found in effective testimony—indeed, they may be the essence of its effectiveness.

In sum, understanding and mastery of the various expert roles described above constitute successful performance of the expert witness's function in the legal system.

Review of Ethical Tensions for the Expert Witness

The expert's ethical universe has been addressed in the precursor volume (4), but some basic points may be reviewed here in brief. Three factors create ethical tension for the expert witness: the role of clinician, the task of the attorney, and the social context.

The role of clinician differs essentially from that of expert witness (5), since clinicians treat, and attempt to help, *patients*, under the guidance of such principles as *primum non nocere* ("as a first priority, do no harm"), medical beneficence, and confidentiality. In contrast, expert witnesses work with *litigants* guided by the principles of honesty and striving for objectivity (Appendix 11–1), truthfulness, justice, and, often, absence of confidentiality, since most litigation is a public procedure. Moreover, participation in litigation by the expert witness may help, but may also harm or have no effect on, the examinee. Experts discharge some of their ethical obligations by warning examinees at the outset of these differences from ordinary clinical work (4).

In following the principles of honesty and striving for objectivity, the expert is even in tension with the retaining attorney, whose role is dictated by the attorney's own ethical code: winning the case for that side. Such a role requires partisan, nonobjective, and tendentious behavior; the attorney, recall, is not under oath. The expert, when testifying, is sworn to tell the truth, which may include facts or opinions harmful to the attorney's side of the case.

Finally, the social context may be a source of ethical tension for the expert. Examples might include testifying on the side of exoneration because of the insanity of a hated defendant accused of a heinous crime in a high-profile criminal case; or pointing out in a civil setting that a defendant was not negligent toward a nevertheless seriously injured plaintiff.

In all these situations the expert is challenged to keep the ethical compass pointing to true north despite the pressures involved (4, 6).

A Central Dilemma in the Search for Truth

In most litigation witnesses are not permitted to speak directly to the credibility of another witness in the case or the believability of another witness's testimony; proscribed support for another witness's testimony is sometimes referred to as *bolstering*. This general principle, though understandable, places the expert in the middle of a nearly insoluble dilemma (7).

On the one hand, the expert is generally not permitted to testify to the credibility of another witness, including an examinee who has been interviewed for a forensic purpose, criminal or civil; to do so is considered to be "invading the province of the fact finder." On the other hand, an expert is obligated to consider the possibility of malingering in nearly every forensic assessment done for *any* purpose: insanity, emotional injury, malpractice, and so on. Indeed, *failure* to consider malingering would constitute substandard practice for the forensic psychiatrist (4, 7).

Since a diagnosis of malingering clearly critiques a party's credibility, the expert appears caught in a quandary when it comes to testifying about the approach employed in reaching the opinion. Experts commonly resolve the problem by avoiding testimony that invades the province of the fact finder (deciding whether malingering is indeed present) and by describing the findings as "consistent with malingering" or using some similar locution or illustration—for example, pointing out discrepancies in the database. Whether this is acceptable may depend more on the attitude of the presiding judge than on statutory factors.

Note for completeness that 1) malingering and its relative, factitious disorder, are legitimate psychiatric diagnoses with current DSM definitions (8), 2) detection of malingering is becoming increasingly scientific and reliable, and 3) malingering should never be an exclusion diagnosis arrived at merely because certain symptoms are or are not present.

Attorney Strategies in Confronting Experts

Evidentiary Limitations

Opposing counsel can limit—even eviscerate—an expert's testimony by invoking evidentiary rules that attempt to exclude the very data on which the expert's opinion rests; some judges will then grant these requests for exclusions. Few experiences are more frustrating for the expert than being prevented from backing up critical points with the relevant data, as shown in the examples below.

Example 1

In a case alleging posttraumatic stress disorder as the result of a trauma, the judge ruled that the expert could not ask about the nature of the traumatic stressor or the litigant's response to that stressor. The expert withdrew from the case.

Example 2

A mother had threatened her children with a knife during an intense episode in a divorce proceeding. In that context she brought a highly suspect claim of child sexual abuse against the father. The expert was prepared to testify about the forensic flaws in the total assessment—flaws that made the claim doubtful. The judge interrupted that testimony to state that he had already made a finding of fact that the abuse had occurred. The expert was left trying to figure out what he was doing in court and to distinguish for the court between legal and clinical facts. This effort failed. The knife-wielding mother obtained custody.

Collateral Sources

Opposing counsel commonly attempts to undermine the credibility and, by implication, the testimony of the expert. For example, the attorney may confront the expert with articles, lectures, and prior testimony in other cases (even radically different cases) in an attempt to show inconsistency and venality, allowing the jury to infer that the expert will say anything for money. In malpractice cases the expert must expect to be asked if he or she has been sued. In divorce cases the expert's marital history may be explored (see Chapter 8 in this volume concerning personal questions asked of experts). With the power of the Internet, adverse information about the expert is sought in police, financial, military, and other databases.

Example 3

On advice from her tax attorney, a woman expert had had a suit filed, in part against herself, on behalf of her children for the purpose of removing a bank co-trustee from the children's trust. At a later trial she was asked if she had ever been sued by her children. She answered yes and began to explain. Opposing counsel cut off her explanation; the retaining attorney's objection was denied. Though the matter was irrelevant to the facts of the case at hand, the jury was left with the impression that the expert was such a loathsome person and mother that even her own children had sued her.

The expert who steers clear of the reefs and shoals noted above may successfully navigate the seas of litigation to serve the legitimate need of the legal system for psychiatric input in many of its deliberations. The remainder of this book further charts that process.

References

1. Brodsky SL: The Expert Expert Witness: More Maxims and Guidelines for Testifying in Court. Washington, DC, American Psychological Association, 1999
2. Simon RI: The psychologically vulnerable witness: an emerging forensic consulting role. J Am Acad Psychiatry Law 29:33–41, 2001
3. Gutheil TG: The presentation of forensic psychiatric evidence in court. Isr J Psychiatry Relat Sci 37:137–144, 2000
4. Gutheil TG: The Psychiatrist as Expert Witness. Washington, DC, American Psychiatric Press, 1998
5. Strasburger LH, Gutheil TG, Brodsky A: On wearing two hats: role conflict in serving as both psychotherapist and expert witness. Am J Psychiatry 154:448–456, 1997
6. Gutheil TG, Simon RI: Attorneys' pressures on the expert witness: early warning signs of endangered honesty, objectivity and fair compensation. J Am Acad Psychiatry Law 27:546–553, 1999
7. Gutheil TG, Sutherland PK: Forensic assessment, witness credibility and the search for truth through expert testimony in the courtroom. J Psychiatry Law 27:289–312, 1999
8. American Psychiatric Association: Diagnostic and Statistical Manual of Mental Disorders, 4th Edition, Text Revision. Washington, DC, American Psychiatric Association, 2000

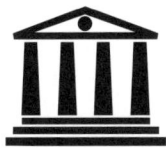

PART II

Practical Matters

2

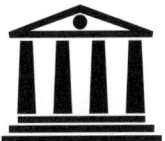

Practical Aspects of the Forensic Examination

The truth, the whole truth, and nothing but the truth...

Traditional language of the oath

Drawing on earlier work and consultative/supervisory experience, we present here areas of difficulty commonly encountered in a central element of forensic practice, the forensic interview (1, 2, 3); these common pitfalls for experts can usually be avoided by preparation and by understanding of the underlying issues.

To review here briefly the main points made in the previous book (3), note that it stressed the importance of allotting sufficient time for the examination in a safe environment, the value of repeated examinations, the problems of third parties and/or recording devices in the examination, the interview rubrics (plausibility, internal and external consistency, existence of an alternate scenario) to which the examiner should attend, the need for warnings as to the nonconfidentiality and the forensic (rather than clinical) nature of the examination), and other details, for review of which the reader is referred to that book.

In the present discussion we attempt to explore the important subject of the forensic interview at the next level of understanding.

The Seduction Hypothesis

One of the most actively debated and central issues in forensic work is the nature of the expert-examinee relationship during the actual forensic examination (see, for example, 4, 5, 6). The problematic aspect of the examination is the convergence of several ethical vectors in one procedure.

First, all good forensic work rests on a sound clinical foundation; good clinicians have the basic skills to make good experts (though clinical knowledge alone, of course, is insufficient). However, clinical skills have a problematic side. Among others, Stone (4, 6) has pointed out the "seductive power of the forensic psychiatrist to induce inappropriate trust in an evaluee"(2, p.18). The paradox alluded to here is that the better clinicians, presumably also the most empathic interviewers, may "seduce" examinees into revelation of self-destructive, incriminating, or other material contradictory to their interests in the case at hand. Indeed, Simon and Wettstein caution:

> The deliberate use of empathy to manipulate the examinee or third-party informants is unprofessional and unethical [citing Shuman (7)]. Forensic psychiatrists who have developed heightened empathic skills from their psychotherapeutic practices must be particularly careful not to misuse this ability in the forensic setting. (2, p. 26)

Second, although all forensic examinations should occur under the rubric of careful warnings about their difference from clinical work (3), the clinical-forensic confusion described above is compounded by the tendency of examinees to slip into a clinical attitude toward the forensic examiner. This may take the form of the examinee—when being asked about personal history—opening up in ways that are insufficiently self-protective for the forensic context. This reaction is especially likely if the examinee has been or is currently in psychotherapy. This tendency to respond incongruously as though in a clinical context is more widespread than it may appear; as Appelbaum and colleagues have pointed out, even research subjects, warned repeatedly that they are participating in research not necessarily aimed at their clinical benefit, persist in referring to the research as "treatment" (8).

Finally, it is a basic requirement that examinees be treated with respect by any expert; yet such respect—though necessary—is itself a "seduction" into good rapport with the examiner and resultant possible disclosure. In fact, the candid and open acknowledgment of the nonclinical nature of the examination that is embodied in the warnings given to the examinee may feel to the latter like a courageous and revealing disclosure by the examiner, which calls for equally revealing disclosure by the examinee—an admittedly subtle but unmistakably seductive element (G. Kaplan, personal communication, 1968, cited in [9]).

Perhaps the most valid approach to these conflicting forces is to remind the examinee repeatedly of the forensic nature of the examination through clear but nondisruptive comments such as "Though we are here for a legal purpose" or "While I am not your therapist." As noted in Chapter 4 in this volume, the contract with the attorney should state clearly that the expert is not practicing clinically in this endeavor. It is also helpful to have 1) the patient's explicit consent to the examination and its purposes and 2) a model consent form for examinees, with an appendix for the attorney's attestations, included below as Appendix 2–1. Omitting this step can have bizarre consequences:

Example 1

An expert witness once inadvertently omitted any mention in a forensic report of the traditional warnings about nonconfidentiality and absence of a doctor-patient relationship. Opposing counsel filed a motion to exclude the testimony because the expert was a "treater." They complained that the report was deficient because—in a supposed effort to simulate a forensic report—no treatment issues were discussed therein.

Forensic Skepticism

In the ordinary run of human interaction, there are few greater insults to our integrity than disbelief in what we state as true. In casual conversations with friends and in most psychotherapy we take what we are told on faith, at least at first. This credulous posture differs from the role of expert (10, 11, 12), which requires, in addition to general skepticism about uncorroborated data, a willingness to consider the possibility of malingering in all forensic examinations as discussed in further detail in Chapter 1 in this volume (13). The expert is thus caught between the general requirement to display respect for examinees and the need to remain skeptical, probing, and persistent in trying to reconcile possible contradictions or challenge implausible claims. The best solutions here are avoidance of affectively charged confrontation and the use instead of tact and gentle but firm persistence of inquiry. The tension described resembles that between narrative truth, which the expert may accept, and historical truth, about which the expert should reserve judgment absent corroboration (14).

The Third-Party Problem

For a variety of reasons, examinees or their attorneys may request that third parties be present in the examination; on other occasions parties or attorneys in the case may request or require that the examination be recorded in some form. One or more of these events may be required by court order, jurisdictional rulings, or other factors.

Certain advantages may accrue from such actions, including the value of taped interviews for training, memory refreshment, or self-review purposes; in more distasteful contexts, tapes may aid in refuting litigants' claims that the expert abused the litigants during the examination. On the other hand, the difficulties posed by these intrusions into the desirable privacy of the forensic examination and the value of resisting them when possible have been outlined in previous explorations of this topic (1, 3). To summarize:

1. These procedures distract the expert from being able to give full empathic attention and close observation to the examinee and, for some experts, inhibit free-ranging inquiry.
2. Inappropriate interruptions and objections, cuing and suggestions from the attorney present may contaminate the process.
3. Examinees commonly play up to the audience or recording device, exaggerating symptoms, focusing on making a recording, or consciously attempting not to contradict what they told the attorney earlier rather than evincing spontaneous (and thus, presumably, more authentic) responses to your inquiries. (3, p. 33)

Certainly, being recorded may constitute pressure on the examiner as well to "perform" well during the examination; although this is not entirely a negative force, it is still a contaminant: the best interviewer is a comfortable interviewer.

In terms of both setting and presence of parties, privacy is the best situation. Efforts should be made to find suitably private settings for an examination to take place; the fact that forensic examinations are generally less confidential than treatment does not mean that the interview should occur where it may be broadcast or overheard (1). If the physical presence of an attorney or paralegal is required by legal ruling, the expert should make clear that the attorney needs to be seated out of direct sight of the examinee and should not verbally interfere with objections and other interruptions. As Simon has expressed it, "The danger is that the consultation room will be turned into a courtroom" (1, p. 18). One attorney has opined that if the opposing attorney has to be present during the examination, the latter's role should be that of "potted plant." While the metaphor is extreme, it does convey the critical requirement of silent noninterference with the interview.

Presence of opposing counsel inevitably makes the interview more adversarial with all the usual constrictions that may bring, even when that attorney is mute. The attorney's presence may render it more difficult to establish a task-oriented relationship with the litigant in order to conduct a fair evaluation. Generally, the litigant may look "worse" or more symptomatic in this situation.

If family is present, the patient may feel more comfortable, become more voluble, and "unload" in the examination. Family support may cause the litigant to look "better" or less symptomatic, also skewing the examination. Under some other circumstances, of course, the presence of family members may heighten tensions, as when family pressures, abuse, or secrets are at stake. These and related pressures may so inhibit the examinee as to vitiate the examination. Examinees often *want* to tell their stories and should be allowed to do so.

If adverse parties are present, it is important for the expert to have an understanding in effect between attorneys that the third party will not testify about the examination.

Critogenic and Contextual Factors

The term *critogenic* (by analogy with *iatrogenic* [15]) refers to emotional stresses or injuries caused by the litigation process itself, even when it is proceeding appropriately. These injurious factors may include such factors as delay, invalidation, adversarialization, and retraumatization through persistent reminders of the original trauma during discovery. As Strasburger notes in an important article on the stresses felt by litigants, "Litigation is not for the faint hearted" (16, p. 206).

The fact that forensic examinations necessarily occur during stressful litigation requires attention to this element of the context of an evaluation. Perhaps the most challenging task in forensic work is separating out the original injuries allegedly caused by the examinee's mental illness (criminal) or by the defendant (civil) from the injuries caused by incarceration itself or by the forceful cross-examination by opposing counsel in a recent deposition.

Failure to pay attention to context constitutes a significant pitfall for the novice expert. Mikkelsen et al. describe a case where every one of multiple examiners in a case of possible child sexual abuse felt compelled to file a separate report to social service authorities (17). At their latest examination the parents were described as "guarded." In this context, where every examiner had reported the family, their guardedness might not be as clinically meaningful as it would be otherwise; yet experts on the case took no cognizance of this contextual factor.

Constraints on the Examination

Attorneys attempting to protect clients or advance their causes may place certain constraints on the examination, either in its parameters, such as time, place, and presence of third parties, or its content—by attempting, for example, to prohibit inquiry into particular subject areas such as past psychiatric history (2). (Note that Chapter 5 in this volume separately discusses how limits on finances affect witness work). For example, an attorney may attempt to allow only a two-hour interview of the client by the opposing expert or to preclude psychological testing. Plaintiffs' attorneys in civil cases may espouse a policy of never permitting their clients to be subject to independent medical examination by the opposing expert, based on the tenable theory that such an examination may only harm their case and never help it.

It may perhaps be obvious that "arbitrary limits placed upon the conduct of the forensic examination by opposing counsel should be resisted" (2, p. 28), but not all constraints may be arbitrary. For example, in suicide malpractice cases or postmortem will contests, the desired examinee may be deceased. Important and even decisive documents may be unavailable or nonexistent. Such nonarbitrary constraints must be factored into the expert's opinion as unavoidable but meaningful influences on the database and data gathering—influences that must be candidly acknowledged.

In all these varying contexts the expert is forced to decide whether particular constraints may, indeed, be factored into the opinion or are so significant that the case must be turned down as undoable. This decision requires close consultation with the retaining attorney, since the expert's decision-making overlaps with trial strategy, the attorney's field.

Examination Sites

Forensic examinations should occur in settings of comfort, privacy, and professionalism. These requirements exclude public areas, noisy jail cells, and—for out-of-state examinations—hotel or motel rooms for obvious reasons. Medical/clinical settings are best. Conference center conference rooms are acceptable as well, as are quiet and private conference rooms at airports. Use of attorneys' offices or conference rooms is more controversial; although privacy can usually (but not always) be arranged, the adversarial context, occasional messiness, and possibility of intrusion may be problematic. In correctional settings, every effort should be made to find a quiet and secluded setting in order to avoid distraction and contamination. Seeking an appropriate setting is an important boundary issue in which the expert must take the lead.

Conclusion and Recommendations

Forensic examinations are an important and sometimes decisive part of expert witness practice. They should take place in privacy with a minimum of intruding or contaminating influences. The expert's attention to contextual factors is essential to preserving the validity of the examination and the conclusions drawn from it.

References

1. Simon RI: "Three's a crowd": the presence of third parties during the forensic psychiatric examination. J Psychiatry Law 27:3–25, 1999
2. Simon RI, Wettstein RM: Toward the development of guidelines for the conduct of forensic psychiatric examinations. J Am Acad Psychiatry Law 25:17–30, 1997
3. Gutheil TG: The Psychiatrist as Expert Witness. Washington, DC, American Psychiatric Press, 1998
4. Stone AA: Law, Psychiatry and Morality. Washington, DC, American Psychiatric Press, 1984
5. Appelbaum PS: The parable of the forensic psychiatrist: ethics and the problem of doing harm. Int J Law Psychiatry 13:249–259, 1990
6. Stone AA: Revisiting the parable: truth without consequences. Int J Law Psychiatry 17:79–97, 1994

7. Shuman DW: The use of empathy in forensic examination. Ethics Behav 3:289–302, 1993
8. Appelbaum PS, Roth LH, Lidz CW, et al: False hopes and best data: consent to research and the therapeutic misconception. Hastings Cent Rep 17:20–24, 1987
9. Gutheil TG, Appelbaum PS: Clinical Handbook of Psychiatry and Law, 3rd Edition. Baltimore, MD, Williams & Wilkins, 2000
10. Strasburger LH, Gutheil TG, Brodsky A: On wearing two hats: role conflict in serving as both psychotherapist and expert witness. Am J Psychiatry 154:448–456, 1997
11. Miller RD: Ethical issues involved in the dual role of treater and evaluator, in Ethical Practice in Psychiatry and the Law. Edited by Rosner R, Weinstock R. New York, Plenum, 1990, pp 129–150
12. Schouten R: Pitfalls of clinical practice: the treating clinician as expert witness. Harv Rev Psychiatry 1:64–65, 1993
13. Gutheil TG, Sutherland PK: Forensic assessment, witness credibility and the search for truth through expert testimony in the courtroom. J Psychiatry Law 27:289–312, 1999
14. Gutheil TG, Simon RI: Clinically based risk management principles for recovered memory cases. Psychiatr Serv 48:1403–1407, 1997
15. Gutheil TG, Bursztajn H, Brodsky A, et al: Preventing "critogenic" harms: minimizing emotional injury from civil litigation. J Psychiatry Law 28:5–18, 2000
16. Strasburger LH: The litigant-patient: mental health consequences of civil litigation. J Am Acad Psychiatry Law 27:203–211, 1999
17. Mikkelsen EJ, Gutheil TG, Emens M: False sexual-abuse allegations by children and adolescents: contextual factors and clinical subtypes. Am J Psychother 46:556–570, 1992

Appendix 2–1

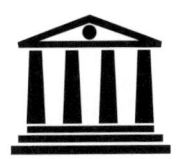

A Model Consent Form

We here offer a model consent form for forensic examinations, which the reader is encouraged to adapt to personal preferences as needed. The model form establishes several important points:

1. The examination is for forensic, not treatment purposes; no doctor-patient relationship should thus be created, and the examinee attests to understanding this fact.
2. The information is nonconfidential.
3. No specific impact on case outcome is claimed or promised.
4. Follow-up interviews may be needed.
5. The examinee's attorney attests to the examinee's competence to proceed with the interview.
6. Very basic language is used throughout.

Thus, in addition to supplementing the verbal cautions and warnings the examiner should give to the examinee before proceeding, the agreement preempts a number of possible subsequent objections and attempts to exclude interview data.

Consent for Forensic Examination

Thomas G. Gutheil, MD. ("Dr. Gutheil")

I, _____, the person who has signed at the bottom of this letter, agree to have an examination by Dr. Thomas Gutheil in connection with my legal case. The examination will consist of one or more personal interviews. Dr. Gutheil has explained to me, and I understand, the following:

1. Dr. Gutheil is a physician and a psychiatrist. I understand, however, that he is not acting as *my* physician or psychiatrist in doing this interview or interviews; I also understand that I am not his patient in connection with or because of this interview or interviews. Dr. Gutheil will not give me any medical or psychiatric treatment, nor will he suggest any treatments to me or for me. During this interview or interviews I will be asked a number of questions about myself, most of which will be very personal. I agree to be interviewed. Dr. Gutheil will explain or has explained to me, and I understand, that I do not have to answer every one of his questions, but if I refuse to give an answer or some answers, I understand that Dr. Gutheil may write that down for the record.

2. Because I am being interviewed in a legal matter, I agree to give up my rights to have Dr. Gutheil keep secret what I tell him. This means that Dr. Gutheil has my permission to talk to people involved in my legal case about the things that he and I discuss and anything he thinks or decides about what we discuss. I also agree to give up any rights I have by law to keep him from saying in court what I tell him or what we discuss. I understand and agree that Dr. Gutheil may talk or write about what we discuss and what he thinks about it in written reports, in spoken depositions (where lawyers ask him questions), or out loud in open court in a trial. I understand and agree that Dr. Gutheil's report(s) may be given to attorneys and/or judges connected with my case as the law allows.

3. Dr. Gutheil will explain or has explained to me and I understand that Dr. Gutheil's written report or out-loud statements for court may help my case, hurt my case, or have no effect on my case that I can see; and I understand that no one can know which one it will be in advance. I understand that I can take breaks if I want to at any time during Dr. Gutheil's interview or interviews.

4. I understand that additional repeat, "follow-up," or "update" interviews with Dr. Gutheil may be needed and agree to them; and I understand they will be part of the same examination and will follow all the above rules.

Signed this_____ day of _____, 200___
PRINT NAME_____
SIGNED_____
WITNESS_____

Statement by examinee's attorney:
I have explained this consent procedure to my client and, by my assessment, he/she appears competent to understand it. I certify that I have answered any questions my client asked about the procedure.

Signed,_____ Attorney for examinee
Print name_____
Date_____

3

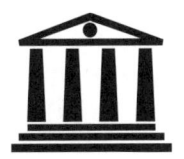

Boundary Issues in Case Preparation With Attorneys

> Selecting an appropriate trial expert is often a time-consuming and painstaking process. As a result, there may be a temptation to shortcut the search by retaining one of "the regulars"—that is, a person with minimally sufficient credentials to qualify as an expert who is willing to say, for example, that the product is defective for whatever reason is suggested by the lawyer who retains her; or, on the other side, that the plaintiff, no matter how badly injured in the accident, is a malingerer. It may be comfortable to use this type of witness, a known quantity who can be counted on to stick to her original testimony when cross-examined, no matter what. But engaging such an expert is often a disservice to the client.
>
> D.R. Suplee and
> M.S. Woodruff, in (1), p. 13

There is a probably apocryphal story heard in psychoanalytic circles that Sigmund Freud would refuse to analyze a patient who left the consulting-room door open on the first visit. He reasoned, the story goes, that this largely unconscious gesture of omission at the very outset of the relationship conveyed that the patient did not care who might overhear the session content; therefore, the patient had nothing of consequence to tell him. Hence, analysis would be a waste of time.

Whether or not the story is accurate, it does convey that first impressions may be determinative, and this is true for the impressions an expert witness and a would-be retaining attorney make on each other. Therefore, we explore this initial encounter to address the pitfalls inherent in it. Subsequently, we describe the boundary issues that arise in the negotiations with attorneys that continue during the attorney-expert relationship.

For the clinician serving as expert, boundary negotiation with attorneys only loosely parallels the same process with patients in clinical settings. In the latter, the clinician sets the boundaries—based on principles of abstinence and neutrality (2, 3)—and bears the responsibility for maintaining them therapeutically as issues arise in the therapy; the patient's psychology usually brings the boundary question forward.

In the litigation context, in contrast, the expert sets certain boundaries with attorneys based on the ethical principles of honesty and striving for objectivity (Appendix 11–1). The attorney's advocacy role is the usual source of boundary questions. Discussion of testimony with advocating attorneys may raise boundary issues that require clarification. It is important to emphasize that the setting of boundaries in dealing with attorneys (especially as regards the content of testimony) is still the responsibility of the expert; often it is the expert who must enunciate the underlying driving principles of honesty and objectivity.

The first awareness that a potential case is out there will usually come to an expert by means of a phone call from an attorney; sometimes, a letter will be the first contact. Less commonly, a notification in either form will come from an insurer or a risk management firm. These early communications begin the process that often determines the future outcome of the expert witness function and the relationship with the retaining agency.

A variety of attorney pressures that may alert the expert to possible problems are detailed in Chapter 5 in this volume; some of these pressures can be identified in that first call. The remainder of this chapter addresses boundary issues that may come up in the discussions that normally take place as the attorney and the expert witness prepare for a case.

Negotiating Schedules

One of the most difficult calculations for the expert witness is the allotment of time for review of a case. If the expert is fortunate enough to have a backlog of cases, the time necessary to review these, as well as time for possible reports, depositions, and trials associated with them, must be considered. Experts are quite familiar with how commonly cases, long dormant, suddenly erupt into action. Even during a case drought, other commitments to job, vacation, and family activities may be on the horizon and require schedule time. Similarly, current case-related activities may occupy the expert for indefinite periods. Further complicating the calculation is the traditional "hurry-up-and-wait" rhythm of the legal system, with its panoply of continuances, postponements, and uncertainties of trial scheduling and duration.

Certain factors may permit some quantification of the time required for expert work. An expert should begin early in his or her career by forming an estimate of the amount of time required to read the various types of documents in a case (e.g., depositions, medical records, police reports) and the time required for performing a reasonably thorough independent medical examination or interview for competence, responsibility, emotional injuries, and the like. For example, if reading a deposition requires an hour for each inch of paper or each hundred pages, the expert can roughly predict the time required by number of deposition inches or pages. As a courtesy, an *estimate* of the total time, if possible to assess, can be shared with the attorney to permit some economic forecasting of the cost of the case.

If the expert's vacation times or other commitments are known in advance, the expert should inform the attorney of them as early as possible to facilitate the attorney's own negotiation with the court system about discovery deadlines and expert availability. Video depositions may represent partial solutions to some scheduling dilemmas, substituting, in emergencies, for trial testimony; however, attorneys tend to prefer live testimony whenever possible.

Experts may be interested in a piece of advice given to attorneys about selecting experts. Suplee and Woodruff suggest the following tips for retaining attorneys:

> How easy or difficult is it to arrange [the initial meeting after case review]? If access to the expert is difficult early in the case, is there any reason to believe it will be less so later?
>
> Did the expert read and digest the materials counsel sent? If not, can the expert be counted on to work hard later when the case is on the line?

What kind of attention does the expert give counsel at the meeting? Are there numerous interruptions for telephone calls and the like? (1, p. 15)

For obvious reasons, these "employment indicators" should be carefully considered by experts in their initial negotiations with attorneys.

Planning for Depositions

Depositions are usually far easier to schedule than trials, since fewer people and shorter time intervals are involved. The deposition, however, constitutes the first time the expert is presented to the opposing side as a witness (rather than as writer of the report that may have preceded deposition). The importance of preparation for this event has been described in the companion volume (4); briefly summarized, the advice given there is to prepare as thoroughly and carefully as for a trial.

This last point about preparation leads to the understanding that depositions may be roughly divided into two main types, with mixtures possible in some cases; the two types may be metaphorically characterized as "poker" and "crusher." Which type the expert attempts to employ is itself a topic of negotiation with the attorney.

As in the card game that is its namesake, the purpose in a poker type of deposition is to conceal one's cards from the opponent. This approach is commonly used when settlement is highly unlikely and going to trial is a foregone conclusion. Here, the attorney has elected to advise the expert to give out minimal information in response to the other side's questions—short, terse answers—as a means of concealing as much as possible whatever trial strategy the attorney plans to use. In this model the expert volunteers nothing. Of course, the expert must still answer the question truthfully—but should answer it austerely, then wait for the next question. If an area is not queried at all, that is the examining attorney's problem. Some experienced experts believe that this austere approach is the *only* type of approach to depositions: one is minimalist at deposition and expansive at trial.

In the crusher model the purpose of the deposition is simply *to promote a settlement* by the conceptual equivalent of force majeure. This is accomplished by a show of strength, in which the expert, at the attorney's bidding, presents *all* the arguments and opinions in the case as persuasively as possible, demonstrating the extensive preparation and mastery of the case that have been achieved in this instance. This complete opinion may even require answers that go beyond the narrow question asked, in order to ensure that the examining attorney feels the full weight of expected testimony.

Experts should be cautioned that they must avoid becoming an extension of the attorney and assuming his or her advocacy position during the above negotiations. The expert's willingness to be guided by the attorney's vision of trial or pretrial strategy should not be confused with willingness to adopt the attorney's legal views of the case.

Preparing and Rehearsing Testimony

The process of discussing actual testimony with an attorney before deposition and/or trial is one of the most complex and ethically sensitive transactions that the expert witness must undertake. The underlying role distinctions reviewed in Chapter 1 in this volume come into play, as an intricate dance takes place between the expert's striving for objectivity and the attorney's commitment to winning the case. Some of the pressures described in Chapter 5 in this volume may be exerted at this point.

Cases that represent extremes—transparent malpractice, obvious incompetence, universally recognized insanity—do not require a great deal of discussion. Only rarely, however, are cases so unambiguous that there is no need for this step. Given this common ambiguity, the expert is challenged to display some flexibility about *how* psychiatric opinions are presented (since, as a part of trial strategy, that is legitimately the attorney's province) *without compromising the core elements that went into those opinions*.

The expert is often pressed to consult his or her own moral compass in this procedure. Is malingering truly a possibility in this case, or is there really no evidence of it, so that ultimately speculation about its possible presence is inappropriately misleading to the jury? Did the defendant's insanity dictate that knowledge of criminality was absent, or was moral wrongfulness present at a high, and less relevant, level of abstraction? How much was this plaintiff actually injured by the defendant's acts, and how much was really traceable to a preexisting condition?

As can immediately be seen from the few examples given above, the discussions here go to the core of the art of forensic work and the related assessment process.

A common dilemma faced by the expert in negotiating with the retaining attorney may be titled "Leaving It to Cross-Examination." The issue takes this form: given that the expert is sworn to tell the whole truth, under what circumstances may the expert present (at deposition or trial) a truthful but terse answer as desired by the retaining attorney, leaving it to the opposing side to bring out the balance of that point?

The ethical problem here goes beyond the expert's ultimate ethical test, honesty on cross-examination (4), since the expert should be willing to answer truthfully all the other side's queries. There are two somewhat conflicting analyses of the matter.

One model holds that once the expert takes the oath, he or she becomes an advocate for truth alone; the expert stands above the legal system's adversarial structure. The answers given are complete and balanced; any qualifiers to the opinion are presented simultaneously with the core opinions.

The second model accepts the fact that the expert is serving the aims of justice by participation in an adversarial proceeding. The expert should present the opinion that has been ethically arrived at both clearly and persuasively. In the adversary system the other side has always had the burden of bringing out the qualifiers, limits, and insufficiencies of the expert's views.

These two models have only one thing in common: the expert's absolute obligation 1) to adhere to honesty and striving for objectivity and 2) to make clear to the retaining attorney what path the expert plans to follow. Surprising your retaining attorney is not good for your mental health.

Participation in Opening Statement and Closing Argument

Closer to trial, additional negotiations between the expert witness and the retaining attorney become important. Under ordinary circumstances the expert should always work actively with the retaining attorney to craft the direct examination in anticipation of trial. Although the occasional attorney's narcissistic resistance to input regrettably makes this impossible, this step is usually essential in order to be certain that the questions are clear to the expert and that the flow of the direct examination will accomplish the requisite task of bringing out the forensic information in an organized manner that can readily be understood by the fact finder. As noted elsewhere, the direct examination should optimally have a theme or "story" to permit understanding by lay audiences (4, 5, 6).

An additional potentially valuable function for the experienced expert is participation in the crafting of the opening statement and closing argument. Collaboration with the attorney regarding the opening statement may be especially important because 1) juries often make their decisions in relatively durable form at the opening-statement phase of a trial and 2) the attorney's preview of what the expert will say should approximate the actual planned testimony. During such consultative collaboration, the expert should, once again, remain mindful of the pitfall that can result if testimony is influenced by an advocacy bias.

Again, to avoid confusion, we must distinguish between the *generic* consulting efforts of the expert and the *specific role function* of the consulting or nontestifying expert, as outlined in Chapter 1 in this volume.

Closing argument commonly includes a summary of the expert's main points; here, again, review with the expert for accuracy may be helpful to all. But closings do not invariably involve summaries of expert witness testimony. The attorney may be attempting to move the case away from the experts on both sides in an effort to engage the jury's emotions, regardless of testimony; attorneys of this persuasion may see experts as canceling each other out rather than contributing to the jury's grasp of a case.

Conclusion

Preparation with one's retaining attorney, in addition to raising the issue of boundaries addressed in this chapter, constitutes the core of an expert's mission to translate clinical concepts into legal terms. Since this is often art rather than science, experience is of enormous value here. The authors hope that the above discussion helps experts to think through the complexities of the subject and arrive at solutions that are both ethically sound and useful to the legal system.

References

1. Suplee DR, Woodruff MS: The pretrial use of experts. Pract Lawyer 33:9–24, 1987
2. Simon RI: Defensive psychiatry and the disruption of treatment boundaries. Isr J Psychiatry Relat Sci 37:124–131, 2000
3. Gutheil TG, Gabbard GO: The concept of boundaries in clinical practice: theoretical and risk management dimensions. Am J Psychiatry 150:188–196, 1993
4. Gutheil TG: The Psychiatrist as Expert Witness. Washington, DC, American Psychiatric Press, 1998

5. Brodsky SL: The Expert Expert Witness: More Guidelines and Maxims for Testifying in Court. Washington, DC, American Psychological Association, 1999
6. Lifson L, Simon RI (eds): The Mental Health Practitioner and the Law: A Comprehensive Handbook. Cambridge, MA, Harvard University Press, 1998

4

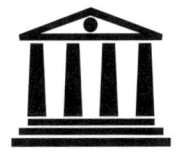

Fee Agreements and Finances in Forensic Practice

Theoretical and Empirical Dimensions

> The expert should obtain a written agreement spelling out compensation expectations and outlining who is responsible for the expert's payment—the attorney or the client. A written agreement will serve to reduce misunderstandings.
>
> ExpertPages.com Newsletter (1)

The predecessor volume, to which the reader is referred, reviews many basic issues about fees and fee setting (2); here we attempt to raise the discussion to the next level.

Attitudes Toward Money

When senior mentors meet with trainees in the forensic field, the first piece of advice handed out is commonly "Get the money up front," or some variation thereof. While the majority of attorneys are efthical and responsible when it comes to paying their retained experts, a disturbing number unfortunately cannot be relied on to behave in the appropriate professional manner. Conflicts about money are, of course, part of the larger human condition and are familiar to clinicians not only from dealing with patients' conflicts but also from working with their own (3, 4).

Money has both intrinsic and extrinsic value. *Extrinsic value* refers to the goods and services that can be purchased with it. *Intrinsic value* refers to the psychological meaning of money, for example, power, autonomy, control, worth, professional competence, winning/losing, and many other personal and symbolic meanings.

To maintain perspective, forensic psychiatrists must understand the intrinsic value that money holds for them, not only because such an understanding aids in controlling bias but because money issues will receive close scrutiny in litigation.

Consider this example from an actual deposition:

> Opposing counsel: Doctor, how much do you charge for patient treatment?
> Expert witness: It varies considerably depending on time and type of treatment.
> OC: Just give me a range.
> EW: Anywhere from $10 to $150 an hour.
> OC: What is your fee in this case?
> EW: $400 an hour.
> OC: That is what you are charging me for this deposition, isn't it Doctor?
> EW: Yes.
> OC: Is that the reason you have decreased your time treating patients and increased your time taking legal cases?
> EW: I get paid for my time, just as you do.

Note that this last response, though true on its face, constitutes an evasive and perhaps defensive answer. The shift in question from clinical to forensic work is quite defensible but may be conflicted as well.

We might generalize to say that the manner in which fee issues are handled with the attorneys involved reflects understanding (or lack thereof) of the extrinsic/intrinsic value that money has for the forensic psychiatrist. Experts do well to consider the ancient saw, "It's only money."

In this chapter we explore the issues of payment for forensic services and the use of fee agreements or contracts to facilitate the process.

Business Aspects of Forensic Work

In addition to its stimulating intellectual challenges and often fascinating clinical aspects, forensic psychiatry is also a way of making a living, with its own business components. As earlier empirical studies of billing practices have noted, the financial aspects of our work are neither often nor readily discussed, perhaps because of unconscious taboos about money and other factors (3, 5, 6).

The usual sources of forensic income for "private practitioners" (that is, those who are not on salary at a particular institution, such as a corrections facility) are attorneys and courts, with the former predominating; thus, most practitioners must enter into business dealings with attorneys and law firms as an inescapable part of their practice.

The majority of those practicing attorneys who retain forensic psychiatrists usually understand and respect the expert witness relationship and regard its attendant fees as legitimate and cost-effective business expenses, an understanding that leads them to pay their invoices appropriately and even promptly; indeed, most attorneys themselves use some form of retainer agreement or contract with clients and are quite comfortable with the concept. But as happens with all professions, forensic practitioners dealing with attorneys have sometimes encountered difficulties in obtaining fair payment for their services (7, 8). These difficulties may be divided into several standard types.

1. *Cash flow problems.*   Especially with plaintiffs' attorneys in smaller firms, the firm's own income may come in slowly and in small volume. This may leave the attorney short on cash to pay the expert in a timely manner. This problem can often be negotiated and various payment plans invoked, but experts must attempt—for their own peace of mind—to obtain as clear a picture as possible about any financial constraints or limitations on their work. The discussion may lead to the expert's rejecting the case, of course. If the case *is* undertaken despite this problem, any limitations on the available data that flow from financial constraints (e.g., inability to arrange for an out-of-state independent medical examination, for instance) may need to be identified from the start. Possible resultant limitations of expert opinions may then be discussed.

A special variant of this problem occurs when an attorney or firm has "bet the farm" on a particular case; i.e., has financially gone out on a limb to a precarious extent to fund its side's preparation of the case; this situation was convincingly portrayed in the recent movie *A Civil Action*. If the case should then go against the firm, the expert may be in straits as dire as those of the attorney, since bankruptcies may follow.

2. *Disorganization.* No intrinsic gift for business management comes along with an attorney's degree. Some attorneys are unable to "get it together" to handle effectively their own financial responsibilities, including expert fees. Those fees may thus be slow in payment. More regrettably, some attorneys plead disorganization as a rationalization for withholding payment.

3. *Narcissistic sense of entitlement and other pathology.* Sometimes the reasons for slow or absent payment owe more to the DSM than to the CPA. Entitlement or, more rarely, outright psychopathology may lead a few attorneys to withhold payment for prolonged periods or indefinitely, so that nothing short of litigation will pry the funds loose. In such cases experts must decide whether the time, nuisance, and effort required to mount a collection effort are worth it in a given case; obviously, the size of the debt may be decisive.

If the amount of the debt is large enough to merit the effort, the collection process should be viewed as consisting of several steps, the milder ones taken first to preserve the relationship as long as possible. Letters to the attorney reminding him or her of the balance should be the first step, and should address the addition of interest charges if those have been specified in the fee agreement. Calling the senior or managing partner of the law firm may have positive effects, since ethical firms do not wish to alienate experts whom they may wish to use in the future. Letters of increasing seriousness may follow, threatening termination of services by a set deadline, which should be adhered to; no further work should be done on the case from this point.

Should use of collection agencies be threatened in the middle of a case? Some experts believe this is a kiss of death, for a number of reasons. First, such threats get attorneys' adversarial juices flowing and may lead them to counter with legal maneuvers. The decision to invoke collection may also reflect the expert's own countertransference issues. A useful prophylaxis may be to make sure the retainer agreement indicates that nonpayment after a specified limit *may* lead to termination of the agreement and expert relationship. Some fee agreements state directly that fee disputes or related legal actions will be brought before the American Arbitration Association or court, at the expert's discretion; such steps should be undertaken after any hopes of resolving the matter have failed.

If all else fails and formal collection after withdrawal from the case is the final resort, an agency should be found that is persistent but not harassing. Choosing an agency that goes directly for the attorney's or firm's credit rating is most effective; indeed, threat of an assault on the credit rating should be included in later dunning letters. Expect to pay the agency up to 40%–50% of what you are owed. If collection fails, small claims court may be the only recourse.

Some caution should be employed in widely distributing the names of chronically defaulting attorneys. While experts can save their friends and colleagues much grief by using such a "hall of shame" listing, the practice comes close to "blackballing" and—if detected by those on the list—may lead to threats of libel or similar claims.

4. *"Contingent" fees.* Contingency fees for attorneys—fees contingent on a successful outcome of the case—are standard practice, usually with plaintiffs' attorneys whose clients may be unable to afford the cost of litigation and who must front the expenses of pursuing a claim. Forensic psychiatrists and physicians, in contrast, are ethically barred from billing on a contingency basis, since that practice is thought to contaminate the objectivity of the expert's opinion and to link the expert inappropriately to the case outcome (Appendix 11–1, Guideline IV, 9). However, venal attorneys may refuse or withhold payment when the expert's opinion, objectively reached though it may be, is not in tune with their own wishes; thus, they treat the cost of expert witness consultation as a "contingency fee": contingent on agreement with their legal posture. This is the most venal form of payment difficulty for the forensic practitioner, since it attempts to corrupt the objectivity of the expert's opinion (7). As outlined below, one of the main functions of a fee agreement is to provide some protection against this problem. The threat of nonpayment for a divergent opinion may be used highly inappropriately as a coercive pressure on the expert witness. This practice is discussed in more detail in Chapter 5 in this volume.

An additional point should be made here. As the authors will attest from personal experience, the refusal to pay an expert legitimately contracted fees is *not* considered unethical conduct for attorneys. This surprising finding appears to owe its basis to the notion that expert fees are purely business expenses, to be handled, if unpaid, through small claims court or similar means. No ethical duty to honor one's agreements with an expert is formally recognized by the bar associations.

This point was brought home quite concretely by two separate attempts to lodge ethics complaints with the boards of bar overseers in two different states. Even when appealed to the review level of the boards, both complaints were dismissed as *not constituting ethics violations* but constituting instead a business practices issue. Both cases, additionally, involved signed fee contracts.

The Use of Fee Agreements

In addition to all the difficulties noted above, experts face the problem of a largely "feast or famine" business rhythm; as one senior practitioner has expressed it, forensic work "is a low-volume, fairly high-dollar 'business,' with very few billing or payment [transactions] and few clients at any given point in time" (W.H. Reid, personal communication, August 1999). Forensic practice is largely unpredictable as to new work, the pace of current work, and the payment for either.

In order to obtain an anchor in these seas of uncertainty surrounding forensic practice, some experts employ fee agreements or contracts in an attempt to gain some measure of control over the payment process (2, 10).

Some General Thoughts About Fee Agreements and Arrangements

1. Retainer agreements are sound documentation of a process of informed consent. The attorney knows what to expect, a step preventing late second-guessing about the initial fee arrangements.
2. A retainer agreement should not reflect obsessive-compulsive problems in the expert: you cannot include and thus anticipate *every* possible contingency. To put this differently, your fee agreement should not resemble an insurance policy or a car rental contract. Attorneys have been known to balk at excessively lengthy fee agreements; moreover, the expert should recognize that such documents can be waved about in open court and used against the expert. While provisions for situations typically encountered by experts should probably be spelled out (e.g., what happens if you clear the time and the examinee doesn't show), an absolute minimum of good faith should be assumed, and simple, unconvoluted language should be used.
3. It is sometimes helpful to estimate roughly the anticipated time and costs after you have scanned the file. Attorneys should also be kept apprized of continuing or unexpected costs as they emerge. Billing should take place at regular intervals, rather than in the form of a single, shocking, massive bill submission after much work has been done; such an ongoing process may aid in minimizing fee disputes.
4. A retainer agreement is a contract, not a guarantee. The agreement may state how fee disputes will be resolved. If a fee dispute does arise, attorneys will attempt to undo the contract by finding ostensible contradictions, supposedly unclear language, etc.
5. Fees in general and fee disputes in particular bristle with counter-

transference components. As with patients, clear and stable fee policies make for good "forensic boundaries" (11).
6. If a case is passed on in mid-career to a second law firm—as may occur, for example, because of a belatedly discovered conflict—the expert should obtain a new signed contract from the new firm.

Empirical Study of Fee Agreements

The results of a preliminary empirical survey of fee agreements and their use by forensic psychiatrists are presented here (12).

Members of the American Academy of Psychiatry and the Law (AAPL), the national forensic psychiatric organization, and members of the Program in Psychiatry and the Law, a think tank and clinical-forensic research unit at Harvard Medical School, were solicited in person and by mailings to submit their fee agreements, with actual fees redacted, for this study. Those participants who did not use formal fee agreements were asked to indicate this. No further attempt was made to select submissions, except that tips were accepted from practitioners referring the solicitants to other practitioners known to use such agreements; those practitioners were expressly solicited for sample fee agreements. Confidentiality was promised, and actual fee amounts were redacted.

This last step had several purposes, one of which was encouragement of candor. A second purpose was the attempt to avoid accusations of "price fixing," such as might cause difficulty with the Federal Trade Commission (FTC). When experts agree (the FTC would say "conspire") to charge the same fees or to raise their fees in concert, the consumer is said to suffer because of the theoretical decrease in free-enterprise competition. This decrease in competition comes under the FTC's jurisdiction. In fact, some legal experts have gone so far as to counsel psychiatric witnesses that if a discussion about fees begins between experts, they should immediately leave the room.

A total of 20 submissions were received, some containing multiple elements. Of the 20, nine practitioners (45%), including some very senior members of AAPL, indicated that they did not use fee agreements. Comments spontaneously provided by these non–agreement users included the following: "Use one if attorney provides one (occasional)"; "I do demand a substantial retainer up front"; "I give my fees verbally to attorneys, they usually put it in the retention letter to confirm my fees."

Contracts submitted by the 11 remaining practitioners revealed the following patterns:

1. *Retainers and advance payments.* Ten out of 11 contracts specified retainers. Two contracts specified estimates of the amount of expected work and/or the cost involved in the case. Some agreements went on to describe the retainer as replenishable, to be supplemented as work progressed.

2. *Standard fees versus different fees for different services.* While this datum was necessarily rendered uncertain because of the rule that actual fees would not be disclosed, it appeared that at least three contracts specified different rates for different activities (review, deposition, or trial); the remainder appeared to employ a standard fee for all activities.

3. *Day rates.* Six contracts mentioned day rates for such activities as travel and court testimony; five did not mention day rates.

4. *Travel.* Travel in the sense of leaving the home state was specifically mentioned in seven of the eleven contracts. Five of the seven appeared to use a special fee rate or a day rate for travel. Four contracts specified a travel retainer as a separate fee.

5. *Expert practice.* Three agreements attempted to describe aspects of the expert's approach to the case. For example, two contracts specified what the expert would find useful to review and what the examinee should be told about an interview. One contract noted the possible need for psychological testing. One contract included the phrase "It is not my intention to distrust you; it is my intention to be compensated for my time."

6. *Level of detail.* This was clearly the most diverse stylistic variable among the fee agreements. The shortest fee agreement took up half of one page in three short paragraphs; the longest was two and a half single-spaced pages of smallish print. Cancellation policies were mentioned in only six agreements; one such agreement specified the time for advance notice of cancellation in terms of Eastern Standard Time, and another offered differential rates for different amounts of advance notice of cancellation. Interest rates to be charged on overdue accounts were explicitly provided in only three contracts. One contract identified items that would *not* be charged for: alcoholic beverages and entertainment. Three agreements discussed why the agreement itself was felt to be necessary.

Discussion

> When you design your own [fee agreement], you will discover that every subordinate clause in each new version will be poured out in blood from your previous failure to anticipate duplicity by some attorney. (2, p. 25)

An old joke defines a conservative as a former liberal who has just been mugged. In a parallel sense one might speculate that the forensic practitioner who is *not* using a fee agreement is one who has not yet been "stiffed" by an attorney. This appears not to be the case, since some practitioners who have long been in practice do not use them.

More to the point, we might speculate that the level of detail in a given contract may reflect the individual practitioner's experiences with reimbursement. Fortunately, as noted at the outset, most attorneys do pay appropriately for the forensic consultations they receive.

Some final points may be noteworthy. Reid recently reviewed the rules in various states regarding out-of-state examinations (13), a point that is addressed in the model fee agreement guidelines in Appendix 4–1 at the end of this chapter. This is clearly an evolving subject, and experts should make themselves aware of the regulations in any state in which they examine or testify.

Abraham Halpern, M.D., has suggested the caveat that if an attorney violates the fee agreement for expert services in a malpractice case, the expert should not take the matter to small claims or similar court until the statute of limitations has run out, lest the attorney argue that a doctor-patient relationship existed with an examinee and attempt to find malpractice in the expert's work (A. Halpern, personal communication, June 1999). This tactic is just one of a myriad of possible vicissitudes that surround the collection of one's expert fee from retaining agencies and individuals. This preliminary survey is intended to aid in designing ethical and clear agreements with our employers with the ultimate goal of improving our practice (14).

References

1. Tips on negotiating expert witness fees. ExpertPages.com Newsletter. Summer 1999, p 4
2. Gutheil TG: The Psychiatrist as Expert Witness. Washington, DC, American Psychiatric Press, 1998
3. Kreuger DW (ed): The Last Taboo: Money as Symbol and Reality in Psychotherapy and Psychoanalysis. New York, Brunner/Mazel, 1986
4. Adler JS, Gutheil TG: Fees in beginning private practice. Psychiatr Ann 7:35–46, 1977
5. Gutheil TG, Slater FE, Commons ML, et al: Expert witness travel dilemmas: a pilot study of billing practices. J Am Acad Psychiatry Law 26:21–26, 1998
6. Gutheil TG, Commons ML, Miller PM: Expert witness billing practices revisited: a pilot study of further data. J Am Acad Psychiatry Law 29:202–206, 2001

7. Gutheil TG, Simon RI: Attorneys' pressures on the expert witness: early warning signs of endangered honesty, objectivity and fair compensation. J Am Acad Psychiatry Law 27:546–533, 1999
8. Musick JL: Collecting payment due. Nation's Business, January 1999, pp 44–46
9. Current Opinions of the Council on Ethical and Judicial Affairs, American Medical Association, Sect. 6.01, 1989
10. Berger SH: Establishing a service agreement, in Establishing a Forensic Psychiatric Practice. Edited by Berger SH. Dunmore, PA, WW Norton, 1997, pp 29–39
11. Simon RI, Wettstein R: Toward the development of guidelines for the conduct of forensic psychiatric evaluation. J Am Acad Psychiatry Law 25:17–30, 1997
12. Gutheil TG: Forensic psychiatrists' fee agreements: a preliminary empirical survey and discussion. J Am Acad Psychiatry Law 28:290–292, 2000
13. Reid WH: Licensure requirements for out-of-state forensic examinations. J Am Acad Psychiatry Law 28:433–437, 2000
14. American Psychiatric Association resource document on peer review of expert testimony. J Am Acad Psychiatry Law 25:359–373, 1997

Appendix 4–1

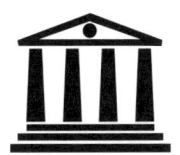

Model Fee Agreement Guidelines

Expert witnesses should follow their own instincts in crafting fee agreements; nevertheless, we offer a checklist of essential points that should be considered for incorporation into such an agreement. Remember that a contract represents an agreement between parties; avoid an adversarial tone.

I. Rates

1. Give your hourly rate; state what it covers (review of materials? travel? reports? conversations/meetings with attorneys?). Should reports be submitted only upon payment of balance due?
2. Decide whether to use a separate rate for depositions, independent medical examinations (IMEs), and/or trials.
3. Consider whether you wish to use a separate day rate for out-of-state travel or a "strict meter"; state any special travel/hotel details. Consider requiring a separate travel retainer.
4. Consider contingency rates for cancellations, no-shows, last-minute postponements, etc.
5. Make clear that your contract and fee agreement are with the attorney, not the client; the attorney, not the client, is responsible for all fees.

6. *Above all,* state your requirement for a retainer of several hours' worth as an advance. We recommend making the retainer nonrefundable and replenishable. A nonrefundable retainer winnows out attorneys whose only goal—rather than to hire you in good faith—is to keep you from working for the other side. If the retainer is refundable, an attorney could send you a retainer and thus keep you from retention by the other side; give you no work to do; then, when the case settles, ask for the money back (fortunately this is rare, but it does occur). You will have lost time, income, and opportunities that you may have had to decline.

A replenishable retainer has you working under prepayment at all times. At times, because of the speed at which a case proceeds or other considerations (e.g., employment by a state bureaucracy) this may not be feasible. As noted earlier, the expert should bill regularly and in a timely fashion to avoid excessive buildup of the unpaid balance and help keep the retaining attorney from getting "forensic sticker shock" from a huge bill.

What if you are given four hours' retainer, and the actual work unexpectedly takes only one hour? Either returning or not returning the excess would be defensible since you had to clear the time anyway; the expert should be flexible with such decisions and discuss them with the attorney.

II. Conditions and consequences

1. Identify the consequences of nonpayment, late payment, unethical behavior by attorney; give interest rates for late payment.
2. Give the conditions under which you might withdraw (e.g., violation of contract); be sure to state that the attorney remains liable for unpaid balances.
3. Consider requiring payment of balances before depositions and/or trials; consider giving pre-event deadlines for payment of balances and/or fees (e.g., "Payment of two hours' fee plus all back balances is required two working days before deposition").

III. Out-of-state work

This comes up only at times but be prepared, since the American Medical Association (AMA) has clouded the issue by deeming forensic work as the practice of medicine, despite the unethical nature of that fusion; the AMA's avowed purpose was to bring forensic testimony under peer review regulation. In some jurisdictions, forensic work may require licensure in the subject state or "consultation to a locally licensed physician." (See also 12, 13.)

1. Ensure that the retaining attorney understands that your forensic work is not the practice of medicine in that no treatment will be provided and no doctor–patient relationship exists.
2. Require the retaining attorney to have made in advance all the arrangements needed to allow you to examine, diagnose, and assess an examinee in that state. Consider following up yourself on whether these arrangements have successfully been made.
3. It is unclear whether video interviews by "telemedicine"—where you remain in the state in which you are licensed and your examinee is interviewed remotely on a teleconferencing hookup—would constitute a way around this problem; the authors know of no case law on this issue. Considerations of liability and admissibility would seem to dictate that such a cross-state interview be treated as though it were an out-of-state interview, as described above.

IV. Special issues

1. If you know your annual vacation time in advance, supply it.
2. Regarding the attorney's signature, note specifically that the signatory shall have the power to bind the firm as well as the individual to the contract; this protects you if the attorney leaves the firm.
3. Consider spelling out a requirement that the attorney supply all relevant documents.
4. Consider explicitly stating that your opinion will be independent of the terms of retention. While this should be staggeringly self-evident, the fee agreement is not only a business contract but also an important informed-consent document, explaining to the attorney how you operate.
5. Leave a place for your own signature and the date.
6. Supply your tax identification number.

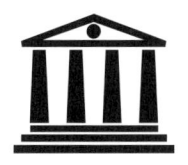

PART III

Problem Areas in Attorney-Expert Relations

5

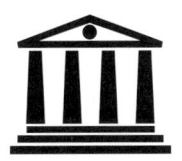

Attorneys' Pressures on the Expert Witness

Early Warning Signs and Empirical Study of Endangered Honesty and Objectivity

> Talking with testifying experts is not like talking with colleagues or co-workers. It is not like ordinary conversation at all. Instead, it is more like the stilted combination of clipped sentences and pantomime employed by characters in movies when they discover their room is bugged.
>
> D.R. Suplee and
> M.S. Woodruff, in (1), p. 65

The goals and the ethical mandates of the psychiatric expert witness and the retaining attorney differ in essential ways—a difference that creates an enduring tension between the parties. The at-

---

With Michael L. Commons and Patrice Miller. This chapter was adapted from Gutheil TG, Simon RI: "Attorney Pressures on the Expert Witness: Early Warning Signs of Endangered Honesty, Objectivity and Fair Compensation." *Journal of the American Academy of Psychiatry and the Law* 27:546–553, 1999. Used with permission.

torney is ethically obligated to embark on zealous, vigorous, and partisan advocacy on behalf of the client. In contrast, the expert is committed to honesty and striving for objectivity (Appendix 11–1, Guideline IV), even when those goals are accomplished at the cost of disappointing the retaining attorney by, in essence, failing to be sufficiently partisan.

In addition, the expert's "normal narcissism"—the wish to perform effectively and make a difference in the matter at hand—is in tension with the fact that the expert is often viewed by the retaining attorney as the "hood ornament on the vehicle of litigation that the attorney drives into court"; the outcome of a case is often predetermined by initial jury selection and demographics, the type of case, the nature of plaintiff and defendant, and the competence of the attorneys, rather than by the expert's skill. Moreover, some attorneys take the position that their need for an expert does not derive from the valuable and specialized instruction the expert may supply, to the benefit of the attorney presenting the case. Rather, some attorneys claim that they retain an expert only because the other side has done so; consequently, the expert is retained because "experts cancel each other out."

The tensions noted above may play themselves out to the detriment of the attorney-expert relationship when an attorney deals with the expert in a manner that either exploits the expert personally (e.g., financially) or exploits the expert's opinion (e.g., by attempting to compromise the expert's honesty and striving for objectivity). Fortunately for all concerned, the majority of attorneys are ethical and honest and use the expert appropriately; alas, some attorneys are neither, and attempt to co-opt, coerce, abuse, or exploit the expert. This regrettable reality brings up the question, how may experts defend themselves appropriately from this second category of attorney and maintain that honesty and striving for objectivity that are part of the expert's ethical code?

For clarity in answering this question, let us begin with an analogy. Consultative experience with sexual misconduct by therapists reveals that overt sexual misconduct is usually preceded by relatively benign boundary crossings followed by boundary violations of incrementally increasing severity (2, 3, 4). Such a progression is referred to as the "slippery slope" of improper practice, leading inexorably downward to perdition in the form of serious harm to the patient and serious deviation from the standard of care. Properly recognized and considered, those early steps of this process can be viewed as a form of early warning system that can be monitored and used by therapists themselves or others to keep a check on the maintenance of proper professional boundaries (5). We suggest that attorneys who initially behave manipulatively, seductively, or coercively toward the expert witnesses they retain may manifest similar early warning signs that permit the expert to avoid such attorneys. Defining and describing these early warning signs may enable forensic experts to practice both more ethically and more circumspectly and to avoid being professionally abused. As the discussion below will make clear, some of these early warning signs may appear even in the initial telephone contact with the attorney.

To take one common example, consider the attorney whose letter confirming retention reads: "This will confirm that you have agreed *to testify as an expert for the defendant.*" This individual should be regarded with suspicion. You are agreeing to case review; your later testimony, if any, will depend solely on what your conclusions are after that process. This attorney appears to be retaining your opinion, not your consultation. If you receive such a letter, immediately send a corrective communication or face devastating cross-examination on a central ethical point. You may also turn down the case, of course.

Sometimes, of course, an attorney's questionable or unethical behavior does not become apparent until the case evolves. Twists and turns in the attorney's case, especially adverse outcomes, may themselves evoke unethical behaviors. Though withdrawal from a case is always an option for the expert convinced of the unethical behavior of the attorney, it is much more difficult to withdraw in the period just before deposition or trial. When the situation is doubtful, the expert is best advised to "play it absolutely straight," i.e., in accord with ethics guidelines, the fee agreement, or both.

A later section of this chapter will present some preliminary empirical research on the actual experience of experts with some of these issues.

Early Warning Signs

The Assumed Opinion

The earliest conversation by telephone with an attorney desirous of hiring the expert may convey the fact that the attorney anticipates what the expert's opinion will be before the expert has seen any of the actual primary data (e.g., records and interviews). This may be conveyed by such remarks in the initial phone call as "So what we need here, Doctor, is the opinion that this person I just told you about is not criminally responsible because of insanity; can you do that for us, Doctor?"

The only possible realistic answer, of course, is "It depends on what I conclude after a thorough evaluation of the entire database." But note that such remarks from the attorney—coming after the expert has received only the attorney's necessarily brief, and almost certainly partisan, phone summary of a case—clearly convey the curious implication that actual clinical data, such as a personal interview of the defendant, are seen as irrelevant to the transaction at hand. A case that begins on this note should probably be turned down.

This problem may be difficult at times to distinguish from legitimate "screening behavior" by a conscientious attorney. Consider the following scenario: An attorney's first query might be "Doctor, this case involves recovery of a repressed memory; do you believe such a thing exists?" Further queries might explore whether the expert's response would be affected by the potential use of suggestive questions, and so on. Escalating disclosures might follow from both sides.

Such "screening" may constitute an attorney's legitimate efforts to avoid paying for, and disclosing information to, an expert who might be ideologically unsympathetic to the case.

Example 1

> In a variation on the theme of assumed opinions, an attorney appeared to be behaving unprofessionally in the initial call to the expert. The attorney, client, and expert belonged to the same minority group. The attorney seemed highly over identified with his client. The attorney's message appeared to be "Here is the report I am going to expect, which you, as a member of this minority group, will surely produce." Note that this conversation preceded any review of data.

Here the attorney's assumption that the expert would give the desired opinion seemed based on the attorney's wish to sweep the expert into his own identification with the client and the client's ethnic identity.

Selected Data

In this situation attorneys provide the expert with only a sampling of the total database (and usually a biased sampling), such as deposition summaries without depositions; some of the records rather than all relevant ones; or only legal documents but not clinical ones. Attorneys may go so far as actually to withhold records themselves ("You really don't need to see the *whole* record, do you, Doctor?") or to urge the expert to skim, skip over, or ignore parts of the database. Complicating the issue is the fact that the expert does not always have sufficient information from whatever *has* been transmitted to know what material has or has not been withheld. Some experts recommend requesting the index to the case file from the attorney to check the list of documents against what has been supplied. However, attorneys may legitimately resist such a request out of concern about revealing the contents of their file to opposing counsel or waiving some privileges, which would allow discovery of work products.

Such withholding may be coupled with the monetary concerns more fully addressed in the next section. The attorney may claim that key documents are withheld to save money that would have to be spent on time for expert review. In some cases such claims of financial constraints may serve as a mere pretext—an attempt to conceal damaging information under cover of budgetary restrictions.

Whatever their basis, such attempts to restrict the expert from obtaining a complete database may well be harbingers of trouble with the attorney. To keep things in perspective, however, recall that experts, for their part, are free to use some discretion as to which data are truly necessary for the opinion; if there are no claims of cognitive impairment from an accident involving a plaintiff at age 60, for example, review of early school records may genuinely not be essential.

Applied Parsimony

Clinicians are well aware of possible psychodynamic conflicts and neurotic behavior regarding money—conflicts to which attorneys are not immune (6; see also Chapter 4 in this volume, on fee agreements and related issues). Of course, overtly psychopathic conduct by attorneys or law firms is relatively rare—though, alas, not unknown. In any case, financial issues may represent pressures on experts, threatening their efforts at honesty and objectivity.

One attorney who "ran out of money" wanted an expert to prepare for the deposition during the deposition itself. He reasoned that opposing counsel would pay for that preparation because it took place on "his nickel" (opposing counsel's fiscal obligation). Such a suggestion should be explicitly rejected, of course, since careful advance preparation and thought, as well as active advance communication with the attorney, are part of the expert's duty in preparing for depositions. As noted by Berg, "Finding out what the expert's opinions are at the deposition is not good for anyone's mental health" (7, p. 10).

Some attorneys have little or no idea of the time required to assess and prepare a forensic case and hence are surprised and dismayed at the appropriate costs thereof; this may be compared to ordering steak on a hamburger budget and then complaining bitterly because the hamburger is not steak. These same attorneys commonly do not trouble to investigate the facts of the matter or to inform themselves about the prevailing expert witness costs in their jurisdiction. For the expert, careful attention should be given to making billing arrangements very clear, and if the attorney shows any hesitation, frank discussions should ensue about estimated costs of the expert's participation. The attorney may ultimately have to be told that he or she cannot afford that expert and a referral should be made. Further discussion of these issues may be found in Chapter 4 in this volume.

In another variation on the attorney-expert dynamic, some attorneys become caught up in a posture of narcissistic entitlement about a case, taking on an attitude captured by the phrase "Expenses be damned, this case is a winner!" This rosy view is maintained until reality belatedly makes itself known when a jury fails to share it. The appropriate remedy here, as in the previous case, is for the expert to discuss just what the finances will involve, or convey this by detailed fee agreement and estimates of time required. This aspect of the transaction may be compared to informed consent in clinical practice (8).

In another case an attorney confronted his client, who was concerned about expenses, with the query: "I can worry about your case, or I can worry about money. Which do you prefer?" Though this forced choice resembles a kind of seeking of consent, it is a false dichotomy; clients should not be forced into such a choice without open discussion of the variables involved. This example further underscores the difficulty that all parties in litigation may have in discussing money issues rationally.

Misinformation or Deception About the Insurance Picture

An attorney falsely stated that the insurance firm defending a case of alleged malpractice could not advance a retainer fee. The expert knew this was false because he was reviewing a different case at the same time for a different branch of the identical insurance firm, where the full retainer was paid without question. This situation underscores the importance of the expert's making sure the attorney understands that he or she is ultimately responsible for payment (see also Chapter 4 in this volume, on fee agreements). The expert should resist being referred to (or fobbed off on) a faceless insurance carrier that is not personally invested in the expert being paid. An added complexity to this issue is the fact that recently a number of insurance companies have folded or gone bankrupt, leaving the expert in some instances holding the (empty) bag.

Signs of outright misrepresentation such as the foregoing are ample grounds for withdrawing from the case.

Crying Poverty

Attorneys may deliberately embark on retention of an expert while intending to avoid, dicker about, attempt to reduce, or otherwise fail to honor financial agreements. Early warning signs include requests for the expert to modify the initial fee agreement or contract.

> ### Example 2
> An expert's fee agreement contained these clear statements: "It is understood and agreed that timely payment for my service and expenses will be solely the responsibility of the attorney, and is in no way contingent upon the outcome of any litigation or settlement. . . . It is understood and agreed that you [the attorney] will pay all out-of-pocket expenses in connection with this matter." At the bottom of the two-page agreement the attorney had typed in the codicil: "Agreed, with the understanding that the obligations of this agreement are those of the client and that neither the undersigned [attorney] nor the law firm are personally responsible for the fees and costs set forth above." Since this clause completely reversed the central contractual point of the agreement, it was understood as an attempt to "de-contract the contract." The expert withdrew.

Attempts to modify contracts in some cases may conceal the attorney's suspicion that he or she actually cannot afford that expert. Rather than seeking a less expensive consultant, however, the attorney plans to use the retained expert and later to dicker about—or, in the worst cases, fail to pay—the fee.

Retainer agreements, when suitably detailed, usually flush these attorneys out of concealment (although not in the example above): generally, once they have been confronted with a fee agreement, they are never heard from again. Experts should demand a retainer fee ("earnest money") on the principle that "if they don't pay sooner, they won't pay later" (9). Retainer agreements serve the valuable function of informed consent documents (see Chapter 4), but, regrettably, some attorneys regularly attempt to vacate retainer contracts in accord with the specious belief that "contracts are made to be broken."

Saying "The Client May Balk"

Ignoring the fact that the contractual tie with the expert is or should be with the retaining attorney (9), attorneys may attempt to disavow responsibility for the expert's fees by claiming that the client may express or has expressed reservations about the contract (as the previous example shows, this maneuver can appear quite early in the negotiations).

Here again the attorney may be signaling indirectly that he or she cannot afford that expert or is either unable or unwilling to honor the agreement.

Example 3

An attorney representing a local client (i.e., one living in the same town as the retained expert) called the expert and said that the client had some concerns about provisions listed in the expert's fee agreement regarding out-of-state travel and overnight stays. The puzzled expert pointed out that those provisions would not even apply to the present case—a local one. The attorney insisted that the client was troubled by those contract elements and was resisting the idea of a retainer. The expert withdrew from the case, noting that if the client could become inflamed by irrelevant and non-applicable contract provisions, and if the attorney took that response seriously without challenging the client's view, working without a retainer would be the height of folly in that case.

The Complaining Response

An issue arising somewhat later in the case is the attorney's response to the expert's initial opinion if it is unfavorable—whether given in response to the prima facie summary over the phone during first telephone contact or after some initial materials review has occurred. Ethical attorneys may respond along these lines: "Yes, I thought you might come down that way, but I owed it to my client to check it out with an expert in the field" or "Slow down, Doctor, I'm writing this down so I can understand it and tell the client."

At this juncture less soundly based attorneys begin to complain, or even to whine: "You guys are so rigid; couldn't you just extend the standard of care to fit this case?" or "Couldn't you just cut the defendant a little slack on this insanity thing?"

Example 4

In an evaluation of an inpatient for dangerousness on behalf of an attorney seeking the patient's discharge, the expert discovered that according to notations earlier in the medical record that had not been mentioned by the retaining attorney, the patient had been described by a recognized expert on dangerousness as "one of the most dangerous patients he had ever seen." When this finding was presented to the attorney, the latter began to whine: "Why do you guys always have to go by the history? Can't you just take my client as he stands, here and now?" Since history is the most relevant factor in dangerousness, the expert withdrew from the case. (9)

The Phantom Expert

This issue is discussed extensively in the next chapter in this volume (Chapter 6) and elsewhere (10) and therefore is not addressed here.

Subtle or Overt Bribery

Attorneys may flatter the expert, admiring the breadth of the expert's knowledge, wisdom, and experience, and saying, "I've got another case for you to work on after we finish this one." An attorney may treat the expert to a meal at an expensive restaurant to "go over a case." Both these approaches can be seen as exerting some psychological pressure, in the form of a seduction, toward a favorable decision by the expert. The remedy is keeping one's own perspective clear, remaining alert to this kind of pressure and—perhaps—turning down even some kindly intended social or other gestures by the attorney; support for this last, seemingly cold position may derive from the fact that a "pure" business relationship is easier to defend on cross-examination as being free from bias.

Subtle Extortion

In this category the attorney withholds some or all payment for expert work at various decision points (written report, deposition, trial) as a means of subtly pressuring the expert to come out with a favorable opinion. The unconscious message here is "If you do not find in my side's favor, you will never see the money for what you have already done or will do." Here again, a clear fee agreement, coupled with the expert's determination to stick to the agreement's conditions, is the best defense.

The analogy with clinical boundary violations that begins the chapter may be worth again employing here. The expert's abstinence and neutrality should be invoked in resisting attorney pressures, just as they are employed in resisting patient pressures to cross boundaries.

Experts' Vulnerabilities to Attorneys' Pressures

Though honest and ethical attorneys remain in the majority, we have focused here on the exceptions to this general rule. We began this chapter with an analogy to boundary violations as preludes to sexual misconduct—a situation in which the therapist's countertransference plays a pivotal role. It may be useful now to discuss some of the quasi-countertransferential dynamics that enter into play from the position of expert witness. What motivations and dynamics on the part of the expert reveal predispositions or vulnerabilities that must be overcome to maintain ethical practice? What conditions might lead an expert to be deaf to early warning signs of unethical behavior by the retaining attorney and thus to collude unknowingly with unethical practice? What are the factors affecting "forensic countertransference"? (Note that this topic is reviewed in more detail in Chapter 7 in this volume.)

The Venal Expert

The venal expert, or "hired gun," constitutes the *bête noire* of forensic work (9). Such experts sell out by charging for testimony rather than for time. The attorneys who hire such experts can be assured of getting the testimony they want (11); hence, for this group, the entire concept of early warning signs is irrelevant: both parties usually know what they are getting.

The Desperate Expert

This situation arises out of financial pressure and neurotic behavior about money on the expert's part. Having, for example, multiple children in college or an expensive house to pay off can induce a range of emotions, such as fear of bankruptcy, the sense of being on the verge of destitution, and the like. This risk is especially salient for the expert limited to a private forensic practice who—lacking a stable source of income on which to fall back—must live from case to case, with income fluctuating as cases are abruptly settled or long deferred. The desperation resulting from such circumstances may lead the expert to ignore early warning signs in order to preserve a hoped-for source of income, no matter how tainted.

Example 5

Due to managed-care pressures a psychiatrist's income from private outpatient practice is severely reduced. He receives a call from an attorney who offers to pay the psychiatrist $1,000 to "review a few records and go to court in a custody dispute case." The attorney tells the psychiatrist that the records "reveal that the mother is a borderline." All the psychiatrist has to do is testify that the mother is "unfit" to take care of her child. No examination of the mother is allowed by the court. During the psychiatrist's cross-examination at trial he is confronted with the American Academy of Psychiatry and the Law ethics guidelines regarding proscription against testimony in custody cases without examination of all the parties, including the children. An ethics complaint is filed against the psychiatrist by the mother and her attorney at the conclusion of the trial.

The Beginning or New Expert

As is the case with any version of the beginner role, the new expert is filled with uncertainty about his or her own worth, merit, skill, and ability. The need for reassurance about these matters may lead inexperienced experts to sign up with any attorneys who appear to manifest approval by retaining them and whose derelictions (and early signs thereof) they do not recognize as such.

Example 6

A very able psychiatrist makes initial forays into forensic practice. An attorney calls, complimenting her on her recent article on sexual harassment and wants to retain her in a sexual harassment case. The attorney says that a retainer agreement is unnecessary even though the psychiatrist's fee is "on the high side." The attorney reassures the psychiatrist that her firm is reliable and will pay her bills. The psychiatrist tries meeting the attorney's increasing demands (time pressures, last-minute schedule changes, additional work, "fee adjustments") without complaint in order to "preserve the relationship" with the attorney. The psychiatrist has long-standing problems handling her own and others' aggression. After the case settles, the psychiatrist submits her bill but is told that the firm will not pay it because her testimony at deposition "led to a lower settlement for their client," compared to some hypothetical amount. In order to avoid any further rancor, the psychiatrist decides not to pursue the matter but to "chalk it up to experience."

The Expert Who Needs to Be Loved

The truism that "therapy works best when it is seen as work rather than love" has its analogy in expert witness practice: the relationship between expert and retaining attorney works best when it represents a business relationship based on mutual respect, rather than a mutual admiration society based on the expert's need for relational or narcissistic gratification. The expert's needs for approval, validation, or support may lead to difficulty detecting signs of venality in the attorney.

Example 7

A director of a managed care organization (MCO) occasionally takes malpractice cases as an expert. He is retained as a standard of care expert by the defense in an alleged negligent discharge/wrongful death suicide case. The defense attorney is a partner in a prestigious law firm. The director, known for brooking no criticism at his MCO, gets along very well with the attorney: they mirror back to each other their mutual admiration. At deposition, opposing counsel takes notice that the director bristles at questions that imply some criticism. At trial under withering cross-examination the expert explodes in rage when opposing counsel points out that "your managed care bias demands early discharge of psychiatric patients, whether they are ready or not, isn't that true, Doctor?" The expert's intemperate reaction markedly undermines his credibility. The jury finds for the plaintiff. The defense attorney is furious with the expert, who, in turn, blames the attorney for not properly preparing him.

The Expert on a Mission

Dietz has addressed the pitfalls of the expert's deviating from the role of forensic scientist into the role of zealot or crusader, whose efforts constitute a personal or political agenda rather than a search for truth (12). The expert with a personal history of traumatic abuse who functions solely to validate alleged victims of trauma, regardless of the data; or the expert who attempts to promote (or to oppose) the principles of libertarianism, feminism, conservatism, right to life, or other agendas through testimony in a given case may ignore warning signs about the attorney in his or her pursuit of the higher crusade.

Here, of course, the goals of honesty and striving for objectivity are compromised from the outset. Personal agendas, if uncorrected, lead to bias and are a pitfall for the ethical expert.

Example 8

A forensic psychiatrist exclusively testifies for plaintiffs. He is eagerly sought after by attorneys in cases involving victimization. His high fees are paid without question. The forensic expert lost both parents and a sister in the Argentine genocide. When testifying, the expert becomes emotional, sometimes even tearful. Juries generally find his testimony very persuasive. Following his powerful testimony in a case of age discrimination, the defense presented undeniable evidence of malingered psychiatric injury. The psychiatrist had not considered the possibility of malingering despite the presence of malingering indicia.

Empirical Study of Attorney Pressures on Expert Witnesses

As noted above, it is likely that the majority of attorneys deal fairly with the experts they retain; however, it is also true that attorneys have at their disposal a number of means by which they may attempt to influence their expert witnesses. Like many other aspects of the attorney-expert relationship, this issue has not been formally studied. In this section we examine additional attorney tactics ostensibly intended to manipulate the expert in the direction of an opinion favorable to the attorney's case. We also describe the first systematic empirical study of this issue, upon which our examination is based (see also 13).

Method

To begin the inquiry, we employed self-report questionnaires given to attendees at a workshop at the annual meeting of the American Academy of Psychiatry and the Law, as well as to members of the Program in Psychiatry and the Law at Harvard Medical School. We hypothesized that respondents would constitute a pool with significant forensic experience. This pool produced a total of 37 questionnaires. Participants were asked 1) to report how often they had experienced a particular practice and 2) to furnish examples. As is the case for all pilot studies with relatively few subjects, the data should be taken as preliminary and—the authors hope—stimulating for future study.

Results

Attempts to Influence the Expert by Withholding Relevant Forensic Information

Busy attorneys have been known to forget to send parts of the case file, especially when the file is large. In addition, attorneys may withhold material that is inadmissible under legal rules or that the attorney does not wish to make available to the other side of the case, as might occur in those jurisdictions where the opposing side is entitled to see anything the expert sees, uses, or relies on. Attorneys may also withhold materials when they honestly believe that the document is not relevant to the expert question being asked.

On the more venal level, however, attorneys may deliberately withhold relevant case material for the simple reason that they wish to influence the expert's opinion by omission, so to speak, or to save money by decreasing expert review time. To explore the issue further, we asked our respondents the following question:

1. Have you experienced attorneys withholding data—either entire documents/records or single facts—from you during the course of retaining you? Please describe with all needed detail.

    After tabulation of results, particularly interesting or provocative written responses were selected; these are supplied below.

    The expected norm for this behavior would be that some attorneys might withhold data for the legitimate reasons noted above, but that *no* attorneys would withhold data that was relevant. If no experts had experienced the latter behavior, the obtained mean would have been 1 (the code given to "no" answers). In fact, nearly half (49%) of the experts responded that attorney withholding of relevant data (specifically illustrated in the comment section of the survey) *had* happened to them, and the mean answer was 1.55 (SD=0.50). This number was significantly different from 1, or a "no" response ($t(32)=17.56$, $P<0.001$). Only 41% said that the behavior in question had never happened to them. (Note that throughout the data summarized in this chapter, approximately 10% of subjects gave no usable answer, apparently based on the fact that they had no experience actually testifying in court.)

The fact that nearly half of the respondents experienced some withholding of data is both surprising and disturbing. This finding might include honest errors, as noted above, but the quoted comments below are consistent with intention on the attorneys' part. (However, we have no specific data as to the motivation of the withholding attorney.)

Sample comments:

Subject #1: I have experienced receiving large amounts of records, only to find that some were missing—deemed "unimportant" by attorney, but actually relevant, if not central.

Subject #29: Yes. Attorney refused to send depositions, claiming he wanted to "reduce costs." I told him I could not work on the case without the appropriate information.

Subject #33: Yes. Prosecutor didn't send me copies of all requested documents; defense attorney sent me none—same case—issue = insanity.

Nonsexual Seduction as an Attorney Influence on the Expert

A long-recognized source of potential bias in one's opinion is that the expert likes, admires, or identifies with the attorney, perhaps even unconsciously; such feelings may lead the expert to slant, shade, or color the opinion rendered in that attorney's favor (see also Chapter 7 in this volume, on forensic countertransference). As with other biases, expert witnesses must strive to remind themselves of these influences and resist them to preserve the objectivity of their opinions.

Some attorneys have been known to try using the above effects consciously and deliberately. We termed such an effort "partisan seduction" and asked respondents the following question:

1. Have you experienced some form of partisan seduction by an attorney apparently aimed at a favorable opinion (taking you out to dinner; praising your work, reputation or writings; indicating that if you find favorably on this case, many others will come your way, etc.)? Please describe with all needed detail.

    Note that the query specifically points to behavior *apparently aimed at a favorable opinion*. This language distinguishes the behavior being explored from that of attorneys who might, say, join an expert for evening dinner on a trip out of state as a courtesy or convenience or to go over trial strategy—common and benign experiences for many experts. Similar points of distinction could be made about offers of future work after an opinion has been rendered, effects of the timing of praise, and so on.

In response to this question, 35% (approximately one-third) reported having experienced such partisan seduction, for a mean response of 1.39, again a number significantly greater than an expected norm of 1 ($t(32)=16.14$, $P<0.001$). A larger number, 54%, had not had this experience.

> Sample comments:
>
> Subject #11: Yes, I was brought into a mass tort case by my malpractice carrier (even though I wasn't being sued) and behind closed doors told I would get paid [for consultation], but we'd have no contract in [the] open.
>
> Subject #2: 1) Taking me out to eat: decline in all circumstances. 2) Praising my work: yes, it happens. I try to remember why they're telling this to me and don't place a lot of value in what they say. 3) I have received hints about future work and view it as a red, red, red flag.

Threats as an Influence on One's Opinion

If the previous query revealed our interest in the use of the carrot, we were also interested in the use of the stick—that is, the use of some threat, or its equivalent, designed to coerce the expert toward an opinion favorable to the attorney. We asked the following question:

1. Have you ever experienced overt or subtle threats from attorneys or

others (e.g., examinees, forensic supervisors) aimed at influencing your opinion? Examples: Attorney will pay your bill only after hearing your opinion; hints that your forensic career in this town will be over unless you come across with desired opinion; threats to complain about you to Board or ethics committee. Please describe with all needed detail.

Note the specificity of language, i.e.,"threats"—which, in the case of supervisors, for example, might readily be distinguished from disagreements or corrective educational efforts, even confrontative ones.

As noted above, the question also addressed the possibility of pressure from the examinee who seeks a particular case outcome and threatens to report the examiner to a sanctioning authority if the evaluation result is unfavorable. In addition, we sought data on whether the distorting influence might derive from supervisory staff. This serious concern stems from off-the-record comments to the authors by some forensic fellows and trainees who described feeling pressured by supervisors or seniors to form their opinions in a certain way, regardless of the trainees' own views on the matter. As the results below indicate, this last issue was not noted to be a problem in this small sample.

Although only 19% of those surveyed reported having experienced threats of this kind (70% had not), and the mean was 1.21, this was still significantly different from an expected value of 1 ($t(32)=16.77$, $P<0.001$). Although it was clear that a minority of respondents experienced this serious attempt to influence their opinions, a result of almost 1 in 5 is still disturbing according to the principle that "any is too many."

Sample comments:

Subject #1: One examinee wrote to media accusing me of sex crimes; [I was] told by attorney: 'That is not how it works,' when [attorney was] told [by me that] I will try to be objective [in my opinion].

Subject #2: Absolutely. The worst scenario (so far) was when a prosecutor stated in writing that if I didn't cooperate with him (I had been retained by the defense), I would never work in my town again.

Subject #29: Yes. An attorney made the underlined threats [to damage respondent's career in home city; to complain about respondent to various professional boards or committees] after a deposition that I handled adequately, but not well. My efforts, nonetheless, gave the attorney necessary information to successfully conclude the case. The attorney then refused to pay for my work.

Ethical Issues

A comprehensive discussion of the ethical issues involved in attorney-expert relations is beyond the scope of this small pilot study, but some comments may be relevant here. The aims of attorney and expert always diverge in one respect: the attorney, as part of his role description, must be unabashedly partisan; the expert strives for objectivity and a nonpartisan position (e.g., by admitting, on cross-examination by the other side, the limits of, or exceptions to, an opinion). Attempts by an attorney to persuade an expert of the validity of one side of a case would be fully legitimate; such efforts can probably be distinguished from the approaches studied here, which involve elements of duplicity and coercion that go beyond simple persuasive efforts and transcend the ethical limits of behavior for attorneys as officers of the court and as professionals.

In a given instance, such distinctions may certainly be difficult and beyond the scope of this self-report study. If a prosecutor, say, threatened to report an expert for violation of a valid ethical standard, the present study would allow that violator to claim pressure on the questionnaire—clearly an example of doubtful validity. A further study might go into the actual context of the claims to achieve more illumination as to their validity.

Clearly, the withholding of data, partisan seduction, and coercion distort and corrupt the ethical nature of the consultative attorney-expert relationship. In addition, these practices violate the professional status of the attorney as an officer of the court, who employs an expert as "consulting educator."

The authors know of no instance where one of these behaviors was made the basis of a complaint to the bar association's regulatory agency. However, while deliberate withholding of data and partisan seduction are difficult to document, the coercion example appears sufficiently unambiguous and unethical to merit such a complaint. Whether that complaint would succeed is unknown. Given the relatively low success rate of complaints to bar associations, constructive disengagement from the case is probably the sovereign remedy here.

Those of us involved in training forensic practitioners owe it to our students to become aware of possible sources of bias such as those described herein and to develop strategies for aiding our trainees and consultees in resisting the pressures that would distort the validity of experts' opinions. The authors hope that this pilot study will stimulate interest in further explorations of this topic.

The Referral Problem

In clinical practice, if for any reason one cannot treat a patient, one can appropriately refer that patient to a reputable colleague who might undertake that task. This common practice poses no particular ethical conflict. But when an expert has decided that an attorney's retention should not be accepted because of signs of attorney venality as described above, what form of referral, if any, is appropriate? Can an attorney viewed as too corrupt to work with you be referred in good faith to a colleague?

Clearly, the expert can simply refuse or resign from the case without any referral at all and leave it to the attorney to fend for himself. In addition, an attorney whose only fault is inadequate resources may be appropriately referred to a younger, hungrier, and less expensive colleague, perhaps a trainee. But if this is not the case, what is the expert's mandate when the rejected attorney asks, "Is there anyone else you can suggest?" "I don't know any other experts" appears a disingenuous answer, while "I wouldn't sully the good will of my friends by giving them your name" seems overly harsh.

This ticklish subject has not been previously addressed in the literature and is rarely discussed in expert gatherings. It appears possible to justify referral to a colleague in good faith if some "informed consent" occurs, whereby the expert tells the colleague frankly of the reason for refusal of the case; the colleague is then free to make an informed and autonomous choice as to whether to take or refuse the case. Referral *without* such disclosure, of course, is inappropriate "sandbagging" of one's professional peers.

Unfortunately, one often does not have the luxury of time to enter into such "consent" discussions with a colleague, since the attorney wants a referral "right now." An argument could also be advanced that an expert need not be engaged in a scouting mission on behalf of the attorney, who has adequate resources available.

A less ambiguous situation occurs when the expert knows from experience in the courtroom that a particular colleague has a higher or lower threshold for determination of insanity, malpractice, or other issues than he or she does. Referral to that colleague would seem relatively appropriate where the case does not meet the expert's own personal threshold for the issue at hand. But if the expert intuits that the attorney is essentially seeking a "hired gun," is it ever permissible to refer that attorney to a colleague whom one believes to be a member of that breed? We would argue that this is not appropriate because, inter alia, it may constitute "enabling" of an unethical attorney.

One might attempt to answer this question with a clinical analogy: one would not refer a patient to a colleague seen as clinically incompetent. But the analogy breaks down: competence as such is not the issue here. Presumably, if such a referral were made, both parties (attorney and expert) would be getting what they wanted. The authors feel that this referral should not be made because it demeans and is bad for the forensic profession as a whole. Attorneys may seek hired guns, but they should not be helped to do so by ethical practitioners.

Discussion

Experience in the field suggests that experts may be subject to diverse influences on their opinions as they strive for honesty and objectivity according to their ethical code (Appendix 11–1, Guideline IV). Some influences on experts may, of course, derive from the expert's own personal history or professional experience, in the form of forensic countertransference (see Chapter 7 in this volume); from factual distortions about a particular case in the media; from professional colleagues as peers or opposing experts; or from the retaining attorneys themselves. In this chapter we have attempted to discuss and study this last source.

Conclusions and Recommendations

The majority of attorneys practice ethically and deal fairly with the expert witnesses they retain. In regard to the unethical minority, however, a number of attorney maneuvers and responses have been outlined in this chapter—responses that telegraph to the knowledgeable expert the likelihood that some trouble, ethical and/or financial, lies ahead. These early warnings should serve to put the expert on the alert for pressures from the would-be retaining attorney that might compromise the expert's honesty and striving for objectivity. Experts may be vulnerable to such pressures for various reasons of their own and may fail to detect or to heed these early warning signs of trouble.

Beyond simply withdrawing from the case—a last resort that may be necessary at times—the expert has a number of options available. Several of these options may be achieved by a clear and detailed fee agreement (9 and Chapter 4 in this volume). Having one's consciousness raised by discussions such as the above and remaining alert to one's own resistance and "blind spots" regarding such signals may also stand the expert in good stead; so will regular consultation with colleagues about this lonely, often isolating work, in which the attorney may be the only nonpatient with whom the expert converses during the work day. Talking with even a corrupt attorney may feel like a kind of refreshing relief from a sensory deprivation experiment.

Finally, the expert should continue striving to identify and control bias emerging from *any* direction, including attorney pressures; only in this manner can ethical practice be preserved.

References

1. Suplee DR, Woodruff MS: Talking with experts. Litigation 19:8–12, 63–65, 1992
2. Gutheil TG, Gabbard GO: The concept of boundaries in clinical practice: theoretical and risk management dimensions. Am J Psychiatry 150:188–196, 1993
3. Epstein RS: Keeping Boundaries: Maintaining Safety and Integrity in the Therapeutic Process. Washington, DC, American Psychiatric Press, 1994
4. Simon RI: Sexual misconduct: how it begins before it happens. Psychiatr Ann 19:104–112, 1989
5. Gutheil TG, Simon RI: Between the chair and the door: boundary issues in the therapeutic "transition zone." Harv Rev Psychiatry 2:336–340, 1995
6. Krueger DW (ed): The Last Taboo: Money as Symbol and Reality in Psychotherapy and Psychoanalysis. New York, Brunner/Mazel, 1986
7. Berg PSD: The great communicators: lawyers and experts. The Testifying Expert 6:3, 10, 1998
8. Simon RI, Wettstein RM: Toward the development of guidelines for the conduct of forensic psychiatric examinations. J Am Acad Psychiatry Law 25:17–30, 1997
9. Gutheil TG: The Psychiatrist as Expert Witness. Washington, DC, American Psychiatric Press, 1998
10. Gutheil TG, Simon RI, Hilliard JT: The "phantom expert": unconsented use of an expert's name/testimony as a legal strategy. J Am Acad Psychiatry Law 29:313–318, 2001
11. Goldstein RL: Hiring the hired guns: lawyers and their psychiatric experts. Legal Studies Forum 9:41–53, 1987
12. Dietz PE: The quest for excellence in forensic psychiatry. J Am Acad Psychiatry Law 24:153–163, 1996
13. Gutheil TG, Commons ML, Miller P: Withholding, seducing and threatening: a pilot study of further attorney pressures on expert witnesses. J Am Acad Psychiatry Law 29:336–339, 2001

6

The Phantom Expert

Use of an Expert's Name or Alleged Testimony Without Consent as a Legal Strategy

Almost any kind of lawsuit is extremely time-consuming. As a result, attorneys' efforts to resolve cases quickly and achieve early settlements are clearly beneficial in terms of both economy and efficiency; such efforts avoid cluttering up the court system and promote constitutional values of prompt justice. Most such approaches by attorneys do not sacrifice ethical considerations in the name of expediency.

Like certain practices discussed in other chapters of this text, however, some of these actions by attorneys steer dangerously close to un-

---

This chapter was adapted from Gutheil TG, Simon RI, Hilliard JT: "The 'Phantom Expert': Unconsented Use of the Expert's Name/Testimony as a Legal Strategy." *Journal of the American Academy of Psychiatry and the Law* 29:313–318, 2001. Used with permission.

ethical practice, and a few actually sail over the brink. This chapter explores one such category of transgressive behavior and suggests responses for the forensic practitioner.

On (fortunately rare) occasions, attorneys may engage in a spectrum of behaviors whereby they name or designate someone as an expert—and sometimes even proffer expected testimony from that person—while omitting one seemingly essential procedural detail: the fact that they have not hired that expert or, indeed, had *any contact* with him or her. This phenomenon, here termed the *phantom expert*, represents a misuse of expert witnesses that raises legal, ethical, and forensic questions.

Examination of this issue leads us back to the most fundamental questions about expert witness objectivity and the relationship between expert and attorney—issues discussed elsewhere in this book. Furthermore, although we focus here on forensic psychiatry, the questions raised here are clearly not limited to that field alone: expert witnesses of every type have been or may be treated in phantom fashion.

Prevalence

The use of experts without their knowledge is common enough to merit exploration and analysis. An informal survey of some members of the American Academy of Psychiatry and the Law, the national forensic psychiatric association, revealed that well-established forensic experts and those who are known for expertise in a narrow subspecialty are particularly vulnerable to such exploitation, on a spectrum of increasing mendacity as described below.

Survey members believed, admittedly on largely anecdotal grounds, that this practice is more common among plaintiffs' attorneys in civil matters, who are in the position of advancing expense monies and thus in a more insecure position financially. However, defense attorneys apparently also use this tactic.

The Spectrum of Phantom Phenomena

Phantom practices appear empirically to run a gamut of scenarios of increasing deceptiveness from the more benign to the clearly malignant.

The Preemptive Strike

An attorney calls an expert and says explicitly, "I am calling you fast/first so that the other side won't get/use you." Here the attorney frankly states a tactical motive. The decision to employ this tactic may be based on the attorney's personal familiarity with that expert, a recommendation from a fellow attorney, the expert's reputation in the legal community, the expert's publications, or a combination of these factors.

Benign Variant

The attorney actually retains the expert, sends the relevant data for review, and pays all appropriate fees.

Malignant Variant

The attorney does nothing further except possibly to claim to the other side that he or she *has* retained that expert. In fact, attorneys rarely admit that they have made this claim to the other side in the situation where their aim is to preempt the expert; however, an expert who knowingly allows himself or herself to be retained *solely* to be removed from a case is acting in an ethically questionable way, since—in the malignant variant—none of the customary expert functions are being, or will be, performed.

The malignant variant above may be fully played out as follows. The attorney calls the expert and does nothing further, but informs the other side: "We have *called* Dr. X" (true) or "We have *retained* Dr. X" (false). The second statement is clearly duplicitous and thus probably unethical.

Empty (Versus Full) Disclosure

Here the attorney retains the expert and supplies the materials but fails to show or tell the expert what will be contained in the expert disclosure, a discovery document summarizing the expert opinions expected to be expressed at trial.

> [The expert disclosure] defines what it is the expert will be prepared to testify to at trial. That description may be based on something the expert said [or has written], something the attorney fantasized, or some peculiar combination of both. However, if the expert only learns for the first time at deposition or trial exactly what it is he is purported to testify about, it can produce some chilling moments. . . . Finding out what the expert's opinions are at the deposition is not good for anyone's mental health. (1, p. 10)

Some attorneys appear to believe that they have sufficient in-depth knowledge of an expert's opinions from a relatively brief initial phone conversation with the expert before any primary data (records, documents, examinations, etc.) have been reviewed; they then base their expert disclosure on this usually theoretical discussion.

"My Name in Vain"

Example 1

A senior insurance claims manager confessed to a well-known and senior expert that he (the manager) regularly used the expert's name to induce early settlement of cases. The manager said he regularly tells the other side that the expert "has been or will be" retained; he often provides the nature and scope of the expert's expected testimony (sight unseen, of course). When asked by the expert to cease and desist from this practice, the manager appeared undissuaded.

The attorney uses a physician's name as the retained expert, and the physician never hears about it. It is sobering to realize that there may be a docket-full of cases "out there" in which one's name and the threat of one's testimony have prompted rapid settlements, yet one knows nothing about it.

Of course, this anecdote alone cannot indicate how widely this strategy is practiced, either by this manager or others.

Example 2

An expert received a subpoena for a deposition—a common occurrence—but was puzzled because he failed to recognize the names of any parties or attorneys in the case. A call to the ostensible deposing attorney revealed that the attorneys on the other side of the case had named him as an expert and disclosed what were ostensibly his opinions, without notifying—much less retaining—him as an expert. Even worse, the ostensible opinions were described in the expert disclosure as partly "based on review of the records" (none of which had been sent). When the phantom expert called the supposed retaining law firm, they rationalized their action as a kind of "place-holding" maneuver. Their aim was to meet discovery deadlines but to allow for amendment of the disclosed opinions (or, presumably, the decision not to use the expert at all) after an *actual* opinion was available. After legal consultation and the realization that bad faith was an infelicitous context in which to begin a business relationship, the expert declined the case and reported the firm to the local bar association ethics committee, without success.

The Part for the Whole

The appropriately retained expert reviews a case and agrees with only *part* of that side's claim; the expert rejects or rebuts another aspect of the claim (the latter constituting a "hole in the case"). The expert suspects (but cannot prove) that the attorney has proffered his or her opinion and reported in a global fashion, "The expert *supports* the case."

This matter leads to the following complex question: how much can an attorney tell an expert about a case before the content of what is told reveals substantive, essential, and protected trial strategy—disclosure that would prevent the expert ethically from working for the other side? This issue is currently being studied empirically. Although this assessment may be difficult to make in an initial "cold call" (i.e., a call out of the blue, without, say, a preceding letter) from a would-be retaining attorney, an expert should, in general, be wary of an attorney who makes "preliminary" detailed disclosures without having retained the expert.

Issues for Forensic Practice

The critical problem in many of the above scenarios flows from the latent implication that the expert's opinion can be known *in advance of review of the data*. As experts are aware, there are only two situations in which an expert's opinion can be known before review of the materials.

The first instance is a fact situation in which the matter is an open-and-shut proposition and so unambiguous that participation by an expert is virtually unnecessary. A hypothetical example might involve a psychiatrist entering a patient's room, noting the patient in the act of hanging himself, and leaving the room after a muttered "Excuse me." Expert consultation to help the attorney define the nuances of negligence in this case would not appear necessary.

The second instance is that of the venal expert, or "hired gun," who sells testimony rather than time and predictably provides what the lawyer wants rather than supplying an objective opinion (2). In this situation, the phantom approach "commodifies" the expert and his or her testimony. The expert is treated as a plug-in module supplying predictable opinions that can be assumed before any facts have been examined. "Support" for this attitude may derive from the potential classification of expert witnesses generally—not just "hired guns"—as plaintiff or defense experts, regardless of the facts. Because some experts do indeed fall into these categories, the attorney may be led to expect favorable opinions from "predictable" experts ahead of time.

For the ethical expert, the objectivity and case-based individuality of his or her opinion represents the core of the expert's value to the ethical attorney and to the legal system. An ethical attorney benefits even by being told by an expert that there is no merit to the case at hand;

valid, important, and economically sound strategic decisions can then be made by the attorney.

Thus, to proffer an expert's opinion in absentia is to impugn that expert's reputation for objectivity, honesty, and ethical practice (Appendix 11–1). Experts' opinions (which vary from case to case) and credibility (which is essential and unchanging) are, arguably, the central—or at least the most important—aspects of their professional standing. They are invaluable and irreplaceable. To misrepresent them is to attack and possibly destroy the ethical expert's reputation and livelihood.

A second effect of the phantom approach is the actual or apparent impact on the expert's objectivity. The specious opinions the venal attorney fabricates and represents as issuing from the phantom expert inevitably constitute a precise blueprint for exactly what the attorney wishes the expert to say. If the expert, against all better judgment, decides to accept the case, his or her views may be contaminated by exposure to this explicit protocol. Even if not contaminated, the expert is clearly vulnerable on cross-examination to the claim that the attorney's blueprint influenced, shaped, or at least biased the expert's striving for objectivity. For short-term benefit, the attorney is in effect supplying the other side with ammunition that can hurt that attorney's case at trial as well as hurting the expert's reputation.

Motives

The phantom expert approach and some of the other scenarios described above appear to have as one prime motivation the wish on the attorney's part to use the reputation of the expert (for specialized knowledge, experience, and effectiveness) as a tactical club designed to beat the other side of the case into submission, particularly in the form of early settlement. This goal is accomplished with great economy, since the expert will presumably remain unpaid (as well as unknowing) throughout the entire procedure. Thus, a second motive would be the simple wish to save money.

In relation to Example 2 above, note that one of the most serious issues for attorneys is missing a filing deadline. This is considered an extremely serious matter and possible grounds for a claim of legal negligence. In this regard, a seminar of appellate judges told one of the authors that an attorney's sexual relationship with a client would qualify as unethical only if the attorney's degree of infatuation caused him to miss a filing deadline!

The serious threat of missing a filing deadline can lead to the following sequence:

In the panic to name an expert [as the deadline approaches but] before the window shuts, especially in the inevitable situation where the expert is not immediately reachable, the attorney, relying on a combination of his or her anxiety, familiarity with the expert and a well-developed sense of denial, names the expert. The expert is then subsequently contacted and, with an embarrassed laugh on the part of the attorney, is informed of his good fortune at having been disclosed. In this context . . . conflicts, [expert] unavailability, [the attorney's] inappropriate extension of [the expert's claimed] areas of expertise, can become significant concerns. (1, p.3)

A Defense of Phantom Practices

A legal scholar and ethicist has suggested that a law firm confronted about the ostensible violation of ethical principles represented by phantom practices might invoke as a defense the notion of precedent, in its legal sense (P. Illingworth, personal communication, October 1996). Under this model the law firm would assert that it had reviewed the expert's trial or deposition testimony in a *previous* case that was fundamentally similar or "identical" to the present one. Such testimony is, of course, available on mainframe databases in several locales and is sometimes used to impeach experts by pointing out inconsistent testimony in ostensibly similar cases. Thus, the law firm would claim that knowledge of the expert's opinion in a substantially parallel fact situation was known sufficiently clearly to allow at least a draft version of opinions to be generated from that earlier event.

This entire concept rests, of course, on the assumption that cases can be sufficiently closely compared with each other *from the forensic psychiatric viewpoint* (as contrasted with precedent based on points of law) to count as similar despite the astonishing breadth of human variability, the complexity of civil and criminal fact situations, and the role of nuance, personal evaluation, and personal emotional response by the expert in forensic psychiatric assessments. It also assumes falsely that an attorney is qualified to assess—again, from a forensic psychiatric viewpoint—when such a close parallel exists.

A variant of the defense noted above is the situation in which attorneys claim that they called the expert and summarized the case over the phone to get the expert's initial reactions. They then claim that this contact (still without any records, depositions, examinations, etc.) gave them enough information to formulate at least tentative opinions for the disclosure. This claim rests on the assumption that an attorney's brief, and almost certainly biased, summary of a case by phone constitutes anything like a valid expert database from from which conclusions can be drawn that meet standards of reasonable medical certainty. Only when the facts closely correspond to the attorney's preliminary account is even that justification tenable.

Note the asymmetry that, ironically, a case as summarized by phone may on its face be specious enough to *turn down* based on its inherent implausibility or flawed clinical reasoninfg, but no engagement to give testimony can be *accepted* without review of primary data, since the details of a case may well include important clinical data whose significance the attorney does not recognize.

Legal Analysis

As a rule most attorneys do not reveal the identity of their experts until it is absolutely necessary to do so; the timing of this event is dictated by the procedural rules of practice. The reason for this approach is the wish to prevent the opposing side from having a "head start" on discovering the expert's background, publications, or areas vulnerable to attack for purposes of impeachment.

Some jurisdictions, such as New York, prevent the expert from being disclosed until the actual trial; from the viewpoint of the opposing side, trial by ambush is the inevitable result. Other jurisdictions operate on the basis of full disclosure of the expert's name, curriculum vitae (CV), relevant publications, forensic reports, statement of opinions, and so on. Under certain circumstances withholding the expert's name until the last moment may keep the other side from deposing one's expert, though the court may still allow this form of discovery belatedly.

In those cases where the attorney engages in some form of misrepresentation (such as occurs in several of the scenarios discussed above), the attorney may be committing both civil and ethical violations. Under common law, "One who appropriates for his own use or benefit the name or likeness of another is subject to liability to the other for invasion of privacy" (3). Each person, therefore, has a right to control the commercial value of his name and likeness and to prevent others from exploiting that value without permission. Courts have consistently held that the unauthorized use of another's name, likeness, *and/or reputation* to promote some business enterprise creates civil liability for the unauthorized user. Although certain protective privileges apply to what participants may say or write in judicial proceedings, a party who knowingly submits false or unauthorized statements to the court certainly risks losing that privilege.

Similarly, attorneys who knowingly misrepresent facts to the court or engage in fraud, deceit, or misrepresentation in a lawsuit are exposed to professional review for possible unethical practice. The expert should inform the attorney committing the infraction of the apparent breach of ethics or civil law and of the expert's intent to seek corrective action. This action may range from simple withdrawal from the case to demands for retraction of the representation or correction of any misrepresentation. In egregious cases (i.e., the "pure" phantom expert scenario, in which the expert is never even contacted), the expert should determine whether a state mandate exists that requires a report to the state bar association and then follow through to ensure that all parties to the litigation, including the court, are informed of the expert's withdrawal from the case or the substitution of a corrected opinion in the case.

In practical terms, invasion of privacy and other civil causes of actions for unauthorized use of one's likeness or reputation may be difficult to prove in sufficient robustness to permit recovery for damages. As discussed in the early sections of this chapter, the attorney has usually had *some*, albeit limited, contact with the expert, a contact serving as the nucleus for the subsequent misrepresentation. The best strategy for the expert is to confront the attorney about the misuse of name and reputation and to demand corrective action, since the attorney is subject to civil redress if the situation is not corrected.

Fortunately, most reputable attorneys do not engage in the practices of misrepresenting experts' opinions or failing to follow through once the expert has been engaged. But when attorneys do engage in such questionable practices, they expose themselves to liability in relation to both the client and the expert; they should be called to task for the betterment and improvement of the judicial system.

Conclusions and Recommendations

1. Phantom practices harm an expert's standing and reputation, the client's welfare, and the legal system itself. Efforts to expose and prevent these practices are highly desirable, though perhaps difficult to achieve. Ironically, rather than precipitating settlement as intended, such practices may actually lead opposing attorneys to pursue full discovery, thus driving up the cost of litigation and prolonging the process.
2. Experts have suggested billing the offending law firm for the use of one's name, charging for keeping a case open, and making other fiscal responses to the phantom problem. These financial strategies

may be legally justified, but they do not address the critical importance of the ethical atmosphere in which the expert and the retaining attorney should work. As noted in the opening case example, electing to work for a person or firm that begins the relationship on such ethically doubtful grounds is probably a dangerous, ill-advised, and self-defeating decision. Also consider that a firm that would not scruple to use an expert without his or her knowledge might well be equally unabashed to default on any debts, no matter how justified.

3. Ethical attorneys, feeling the pressure of time, may at times *ask* the expert for permission to present to the court a "preliminary" opinion (i.e., one reached prior to detailed case review) with a proviso about possible later amendments. Although this request is closer to an "informed consent" model and thus better than phantom situations, in light of the importance of the expert's credibility, in many cases such an offer should probably be refused. It might properly be accepted where the expert has knowledge of, and confidence in, the attorney's competence in litigation of the kind at issue, in which case the proposed opinions are more likely to be clinically valid. Nevertheless, it may still be preferable to refer the case to an expert who can perform an immediate review in order to present a substantiated opinion to the court.

4. If an expert receives case materials, but no further retaining steps or communications transpire despite the expert's efforts, after a certain amount of time the expert may write to the attorney stating that unless the expert hears from the attorney by a specified date the case materials will be returned unread, and the expert will formally withdraw; after the deadline, this plan should be put into effect. Some experts state in their cover letters that this ultimate withdrawal—if occurring before case data or trial strategy have been revealed—does not ethically preclude retention by the other side, as long as the expert makes clear that the case material is unread. Actively *soliciting* such employment from the other side, however, is ethically more ambiguous and should probably be avoided.

5. The expert may wish to consider the pros and cons of reporting such attorneys or firms to the local disciplinary authority for ethical violations. This course of action may have some deterrent effect against future abuses, though empirical data on this point are rare and not very encouraging.

6. For completeness note that phantom conduct can be distinguished from the following common situation. The attorney discusses the case with the expert, who has read relevant and sufficient material. Based on this discussion, a general opinion about the expert's testi-

mony is then proffered by the attorney. This opinion can be modified, as is always the case, if further information becomes available. It is essential, however, that the expert review *any written opinion* purporting to represent his or her views. Here, the attorney's proffer is based on the expert's reasonable review of the data and the expert's direct expression of an opinion based on those data.
7. Based on the legal analysis outlined earlier in this chapter, there appear to be grounds for civil litigation against the offending lawyer or firm. The basis for such action may vary according to the locale, the professional environment, the costs and benefits of the consequences in a particular case, and determination of whether phantom behavior is a repeated or habitual practice by the lawyer or the firm. Although the harm to the expert's reputation is, in one sense, obvious, demonstrating concrete or quantifiable effects may prove difficult. On the other hand, the misappropriation of the expert's reputation may be considered theft of a valuable asset and hence may call for litigation.
8. Finally, this problem should receive research attention, open discussion in forensic and legal fora, and presentation in the literature, as in this chapter.

References

1. Berg PSD: The great communicators: lawyers and experts. The Testifying Expert 6:3, 10, 1998
2. Gutheil TG: The Psychiatrist as Expert Witness. Washington, DC, American Psychiatric Press, 1998
3. Restatement of Torts, 2nd

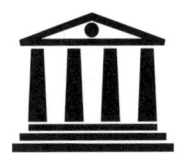

PART IV

Forensic Countertransference

7

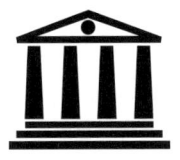

Issues in Forensic Countertransference

Early Warning Signs of Compromised Distance and Objectivity

The subject of countertransference has received needed attention in the clinical setting, usually relating to longer-term, exploratory psychotherapy; a recent joke suggests that one "benefit" of managed care is that under its financial constraints no therapy will continue long enough for countertransference problems to develop.

With a few valuable exceptions, however (1–7), the subject of countertransference in the *forensic* setting has been far less discussed. Bias in forensic practice may constitute the closest analogy to traditional countertransference in clinical work. Clinical countertransference cannot be entirely eliminated, but efforts should be made to identify and manage it. Similarly, although bias cannot be entirely eliminated from forensic psychiatry, practitioners should attempt to identify and minimize the effects of "normal" bias as a natural part of striving for objectivity.

Example 1

A close family member of an expert witness received a distressing and serious head injury; shortly afterward, the expert was asked to consult on a case involving a serious head injury. Recognizing the obvious potential for significant bias, he passed on the case (L. H. Strasburger, personal communication, June 2001).

Forensic countertransference may also have positive effects. Clearly, it is not a problem if the expert can identify it as a form of bias and even use it to benefit the evaluation. For example, the examiner's anxiety responses may illuminate what people around the examinee were feeling during emotionally tense situations associated with the alleged crime or injury.

The expert witness may thus benefit from a discussion of forensic countertransference, which can alert him or her to the potential for unintentionally compromising the objectivity required for forensic testimony. This chapter explores some of the issues related to this concept.

Comparisons With the Clinical Context

Over the decades, countertransference has developed two related definitions in the clinical context (8). One definition, originating from Freud's early work and continuing to the present, is that the therapist's countertransference is an unconscious response to the patient's transference (9). That is, the therapist's subliminal awareness of the feelings and attitudes unconsciously imputed to him or her by the patient (transference) is thought to evoke a complementary unconscious response in the therapist (countertransference)—a response that may draw as well upon the therapist's own past object relationships. Under this model the difference between transference and countertransference is essentially one of vector: transference toward the therapist, countertransference from the therapist.

A second definition, with variations of its own, is that countertransference is the therapist's usually unconscious—but sometimes quite conscious—response to the patient's *overt behavior*. Examples might include anger, conscious or unconscious (evoked by the patient's sadism, manipulation, demeaning manner, and the like), or avoidance of the patient's affective material because of the therapist's fear, disgust, or judgmental attitudes. Under a looser definition of countertransference, the anger example above would be considered independent of whether the therapist had any past experiences with a sadistic, manipulative, or demeaning parent or other early object.

Note that countertransference has acquired a pejorative connotation and is sometimes used as if equivalent to disliking the patient or examinee; of course, positive countertransference, as discussed below, is equally possible and may comparably affect expert objectivity.

In forensic practice the examiner may develop all of the above reactions toward the examinee, who may occupy a patientlike position in the dyad, as far as affective interaction with the examiner goes. Responses to the examinee may follow patterns similar to those in the clinical situation, though often colored by the litigative context, the occasional horrendous facts of a crime, or the personality disorder of the examinee, as seen in the example below.

Example 2

Sattar (P. Sattar, "Countering Countertransference: A Forensic Trainee's Dilemma," unpublished manuscript, 2000) has courageously described the reactions of a trainee examining a defendant for criminal nonresponsibility on a charge of strangling a 1-year-old infant. Sattar notes: "As [the trainee] read the details of the police and witness accounts, he could not help feeling enraged. Being [himself] the father of a one-year-old infant, he could identify with the mother of the victim. 'How could [the defendant] do this,' he thought. 'No man should get away with this'" (p.3).

Sattar goes on to describe feeling tempted to dismiss his largely uncooperative examinee with minimal evaluation, considering him a psychopath. He was able eventually to overcome this countertransferential bias and perform a valid assessment, revealing the defendant's significant mental disorder at the time of the alleged act. The case example dramatically reveals, however, how horror at the alleged crime and a personalized identification with one of the parties may threaten to distort the objectivity required by forensic assessment.

A novel countertransferential response may occur in forensic work, however, that has no exact analogue in clinical work: a countertransference response to the attorneys in the case. Usually such responses involve the retaining attorney, but, under certain circumstances, the opposing attorney may also be the object of such feelings (for example, in deposition).

Reactions to attorneys may partake of the duality noted above: the expert's reaction may be based on conscious or unconscious responses to the attorney's transference to the expert and/or the attorney's overt behavior or personality. These reactions are meaningful for our consideration insofar as they may impair the expert's objectivity in the case.

The following discussion explores both vectors of forensic countertransference: examinee-centered and attorney-centered.

Examinee-Centered Countertransference

Preoccupation With the Examinee

Clinicians familiar with the problem of boundary violations have identified one of the warning signs of a developing potential for exploitation of the patient: a therapist thinking or ruminating excessively about the patient between sessions and having fantasies about him or her as well (10). A parallel experience with equally valuable predictive power may occur in forensic work, where the expert witness becomes preoccupied with the examinee after the evaluation is over or at other points during the discovery process. Such a preoccupation may have both positive and negative valences.

In the positive version, the examiner may overidentify with the examinee's situation and lose objectivity, taking on an advocacy role. On the negative side, the examiner may feel repelled by the examinee in some way and experience fantasies of violence from or toward that examinee.

Example 3

> After an evaluation, a forensic trainee reported having nightmares about being stalked by a defendant-examinee charged with a sadistic murder but was able to work through these responses in supervision and personal therapy.

Not all responses can be managed in this way. Experts who find themselves succumbing to emotional responses may reach a point where they must withdraw from a case because of total loss of objectivity. Consultation is critically important in these situations, since withdrawal from a case is a serious step and not to be taken lightly. On the other hand, serious compromise of one's capacity to work effectively is a legitimate basis for transferring the case, as it may be in a clinical context.

Secondary Posttraumatic Stress Disorder Symptoms in the Examiner

Although forensic examinations are usually relatively short compared to long-term therapy, they may be no less powerful for their brevity; an examinee may yet have a profound emotional effect on the examiner. In a criminal context, this effect may derive from the horrifying details of an examinee's crime; in a civil setting, it may be caused by distressing descriptions of trauma in its various forms. Some sources of emotional impact would be stressful for anyone, while others may resonate in particular with the examiner's personal history.

The trauma literature has described this phenomenon as "secondary posttraumatic stress disorder" ("secondary PTSD"), in which the vicarious experience of hearing trauma-related material may afflict the interviewer with the entire panoply of traumatic symptomatology (11); usually, however, only some symptoms, rather than the entire syndrome, are present. Consequent avoidance responses may constitute a special case of forensic countertransference, leading to impairment of the assessment process through distancing and compromised objectivity, as in the following case example:

Example 4

> A forensic psychiatrist who was sexually and physically abused as a child found that evaluating therapist-patient abuse was very troubling for her. The psychiatrist would overidentify with the plaintiff, who often had also been sexually abused as a child, and would even experience flashbacks of her own childhood abuse, as well as anxiety, insomnia, and anorexia for a few weeks following the examination. She decided not to accept cases of abuse because of this upset and consequent loss of objectivity.

Rather than arising de novo, most cases of so-called "secondary PTSD" in forensic examinations are likely to represent exacerbations of previous personal traumata in the expert's life. The examination of a claimant with a history congruent to the expert's own triggers an evocation of the examiner's traumatic experiences and symptoms. As is true with patients, all forensic psychiatrists have limitations and blind spots in respect to certain litigants. As is also true with clinical work, thoughtful reflection and self-scrutiny constitute "countertransference hygiene" in forensic practice; preemptive recognition of one's limitations is far more desirable than having them pointed out at trial by opposing counsel.

Overimmersion in the Examinee's World View

The forensic evaluator maintains an objective, even skeptical posture in relation to all data in a case, including the examinee's interview data. In some circumstances the examinee may be highly persuasive and convincing, such that the examiner becomes inappropriately immersed in the examinee's view of the situation under consideration. Although willingness to enter into empathic engagement with an examinee is a perfectly acceptable and useful interview approach, the examiner must be equally willing to step back and weigh the material skeptically, as well as comparing it to other data in the case. For example, in an insanity evaluation, the examiner should attempt to become attuned to the defendant's state of mind at the time of the alleged act; but to conclude, for example, "He's right; those people *did* need killing" would be to carry empathy too far. Many other examples suggest themselves as well.

Perhaps the most common biasing factor that may contribute to empathy becoming a problem rather than an advantage is the view of the examinee as a patient. We have been trained to help and take care of people in our therapeutic roles; these caretaking impulses may intrude inappropriately into the forensic relationship. As is true in treatment as well, overprotectiveness toward examinees may represent a reaction formation against sadistic/aggressive feelings on the part of the examiner that may be stirred up by the forensic context.

Attorney-Centered Countertransference

Personal Conflict With the Attorney

Like people in general, some attorneys may be difficult to deal with. One hopes for at least a professional relationship with one's retaining attorney, even a friendly one; indeed, this is usually the case. But law schools, like other professional training settings (medical school, divinity school), tend to screen for the presence of competence rather than for the absence of personality or character disorders. Consequently, an expert may be retained by an attorney who—while initially amicable enough—later relates to the expert in a manner that may cause conflict.

In the ordinary run of forensic work, the expert strives for honesty and objectivity; this mandate presumably includes attempting to keep any personal feelings toward the attorney from spilling over to contaminate the case at hand. However, conflict between the expert and the attorney could reach a level sufficient to justify the expert's withdrawal from the case in progress, rather than merely a resolve never to work with that attorney again.

A different dynamic may apply when the expert ends up arguing with the attorney about the case *outcome*, rather than about the opinion or its basis (the latter being legitimate subjects for discussion, if not argument). The outcome, of course, is the province of the fact finder and is not the expert's problem. Finding oneself unduly concerned with the case outcome may constitute an early warning sign for the expert—one that points to impaired objectivity.

Personal conflict with attorneys can arise around billing arrangements involved in retention of the expert. Indeed, countertransference reactions may be strongly fomented by issues surrounding the subject of money. Stereotypes of attorneys aside, the ease with which financial disagreements can evoke countertransference responses is a powerful argument in favor of explicit fee agreements that pin down the fiscal contract between expert and attorney (see Chapter 4 in this volume).

Overidentification With and Overacceptance of the Attorney

A different kind of countertransference pitfall is possible when the expert has enjoyed a good working relationship with the attorney for any reason, perhaps because the attorney is friendly and personable, or because the expert has been retained by the same attorney on several cases. This is the problem of overidentification with the attorney's position or side of the case—rather than objectively maintaining one's own opinion (12). This positive countertransference dynamic may compromise objectivity.

Overidentification may lead on occasion to a temptation to slant (and thus distort) the data on the expert's side of the case. The associated overcommitment to the process and attempts to "win" for one's side may also derive from the expert's normal narcissism (or, in worst cases, grandiosity), which may distract him or her from the actual challenge of adhering to truth-telling under adverse pressures. As a result of overidentification, the expert may also fail to bring to bear the requisite skepticism with regard to the claims of a retaining attorney with whom he or she has a good relationship.

Another aspect of the expert-attorney relationship that may distort objectivity is an expert's need to be loved by others, perhaps including the retaining attorney or even the opposing one. This countertransference problem may lead to an inability to disappoint the attorney by revealing the weaknesses in the case or by disagreeing with him or her—potentially serious flaws in expert function. Like good therapy, expert witness practice is better viewed as work than love.

To deal with these pitfalls, the expert should take note of a positive relationship with the attorney and enjoy it for its own sake, but then scrutinize the data from a deliberately skeptical perspective. Difficult though this may sometimes be, the expert's loyalty must ultimately be to the truth of the testimony to be delivered.

Defensiveness

Another internal clue to a forensic countertransference problem is finding oneself acting defensively in dealing with the retaining attorney.

The expert is supposed to reach an opinion in a reasonable manner and to review or examine all sources of data considered important and relevant to that opinion. If the attorney questions the expert's interpretation of a finding or omission of a document or data source, the expert's task remains that of educating the attorney by providing whatever explanations are needed. If the attorney is calling attention to an overlooked point in the data, the expert should be grateful for this assistance. Waxing defensive, in contrast, suggests that objective, collaborative work is no longer the expert's main focus. The expert should reflect on why the matter has stimulated a defensive response, which is personal and narcissistic rather than professional. The expert's narcissism can sometimes be muted by considering that the expert is a mere hood ornament on the vehicle of litigation that the attorney drives to court.

Contextual Factors

Litigation itself produces striking distortions and fantasies about claimants. For example, well before an examination actually takes place, both examiner and examinee already have intense transferences toward each other. In contrast to our situation vis-à-vis our patients, we possess a great deal of information about the claimant, as the latter does about us—although this information is usually or even always incorrect. The transference is thus formed in advance and may become incendiary even before the face-to-face encounter because of the hotly contested nature of the case.

In litigation the mutual hostility of attorneys toward each other may spill over to infect all parties, a phenomenon captured in the theatrical drama *Child's Play*. Transference aroused in the litigant by prior encounters (e.g., depositions) with an expert's retaining attorney (i.e., the litigant's opposing counsel) may further intensify negative feelings toward the expert, to which the latter may consciously or unconsciously respond.

Example 5

A female litigant in a sexual harassment suit recoiled when the male examiner put out a hand for a handshake at first meeting. The litigant later charged the examiner with sexual misconduct.

At times litigants are accompanied into the examination itself by their attorneys (13, 14). This creates a grouping that may both diffuse and confuse countertransference factors, as can recording devices in the examination. Being observed or recorded may stir up conflicts about exposure in the litigant and in the examiner.

Finally, litigants have powerful conscious and unconscious drives in the litigation process and comparably powerful reasons to view the examiner as rescuer/savior or persecutor/devil; serious matters of money, reputation, imprisonment, validation, revenge, and other issues may be at stake in the litigation. The intense affective content associated with these issues may clearly evoke responses in the examiner.

Conclusion

Forensic work may be influenced by considerations resembling clinical countertransference, with the attorney-expert relationship serving as a novel source of countertransference responses. This chapter has addressed some forms of this response and some early warning signs of its presence. The difficulty it poses for forensic work consists of excessive distancing from the work at hand and impairment of needed objectivity.

The remedies for the problem derive from the historically validated standbys of peer consultation, personal reflection, self-scrutiny, and personal therapy. The content of this chapter has been predicated upon the principle that awareness of the areas in which potential countertransference difficulties may appear is the first and best step toward remedying the problem. Under some circumstances the time-tested methods noted above may fail, and withdrawal from the case may prove the only way to preserve the integrity of the forensic process.

References

1. Weiss JM: Some reflections on countertransference in the treatment of criminals. Psychiatry 61:172–177, 1998
2. Schetky DH, Colbach EM: Countertransference on the witness stand: a flight from self? Bull Am Acad Psychiatry Law 10:115–122, 1982
3. Protter B, Travin S: The significance of countertransference and related issues in a multi-service court clinic. Bull Am Acad Psychiatry Law 11:223–230, 1983
4. Mellman LA: Countertransference in court interpreters. Bull Am Acad Psychiatry Law 23:467–471, 1995
5. Gorman WF: Are there impartial expert witnesses? Bull Am Acad Psychiatry Law 11:379–382, 1983
6. Simon RI: The credible forensic psychiatric examination in sexual harassment cases. Psychiatr Ann 26:139–148, 1996

7. Diamond BL: The fallacy of the impartial expert. Archives of Criminal Psychodynamics 3:221–236, 1959
8. Gutheil TG: Countertransference, in The Social Science Encyclopedia. Edited by Kuper A, Kuper J. London, Routledge & Kegan Paul, 1984
9. Freud S: Future Prospects of Psychoanalytic Theory (1910), in The Standard Edition of the Complete Psychological Works of Sigmund Freud, Vol 11. Translated and edited by Strachey J. London, Hogarth Press, 1962, pp 139–157
10. Epstein RS, Simon RI: The exploitation index: an early warning indicator of boundary violations in psychotherapy. Bull Menninger Clin 54:450–463, 1990
11. Valent P: Survival strategies: a framework for understanding secondary traumatic stress and coping in helpers, in Compassion Fatigue: Coping with Secondary Traumatic Stress in Those Who Treat the Traumatized. Edited by Figley CR. New York, Brunner/Mazel, 1995, pp 21–50
12. Gutheil TG: The Psychiatrist as Expert Witness. Washington, DC, American Psychiatric Press, 1998
13. Simon RI, Wettstein RM: Toward the development of guidelines for the conduct of forensic psychiatric examinations. J Am Acad Psychiatry Law 25:17–30, 1997
14. Simon RI: "Three's a crowd:" the presence of third parties during the forensic psychiatric examination. J Psychiatry Law 24:3–25, 1996

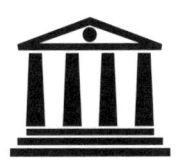

PART V

Problems With Deposition and Trial Testimony

8

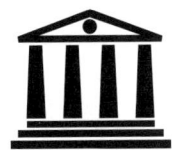

Personal Questions on Cross-Examination

A Pilot Study of Expert Witness Attitudes

> In most courts, expert witnesses can reasonably expect to be treated with respect and with minimal inquiry into their personal lives. Now and then, an attorney who is naturally intrusive, who is desperate, or who has an important case will pry into personal elements in the backgrounds of the witnesses. At their worst, these instances touch on acutely sensitive topics.
>
> S.L. Brodsky, in (1), p. 149

> Testifying in court is lecturing under combat conditions.
>
> Emmanuel Tanay, M.D.
> (personal communication, 1999)

This chapter was adapted from Gutheil TG, Commons ML, Miller PM: "Personal Questions on Cross-Examination: A Pilot Study of Expert Witness Attitudes." *Journal of the American Academy of Psychiatry and the Law* 29:85–88, 2001. Used with permission.

Expert witnesses have long recognized the various challenges to one's equanimity, confidence, and even self-esteem presented by cross-examination. Indeed, anyone willing to testify in court—expert or not—must naturally expect and prepare for vigorous attempts at impeachment by the opposing attorney.

Attorneys, for their own part, have devoted much of their training—and devote, with each trial, much preparation—to their role in cross-examination, in the service of impeaching, discrediting, and invalidating testimony opposed to their side of the case. They are allowed wide latitude, both in what they may ask the expert and on what sources of information they may draw in discovering or designing refutations of and contradictions to the expert's testimony.

In actual forensic practice, attorneys have been known to ask questions of the expert that are or seem highly personal and intrusive, and of dubious relevance to the matter at hand; when this occurs, experts commonly feel that their privacy is being invaded, or that the goal of an intrusive line of inquiry is to create subjective discomfort in the witness rather than to present persuasive data to the jury. It may be helpful to the expert, however, to realize that personal questions arise, for the most part, from the attorney's ethical duty to provide zealous advocacy for his or her client. Put another way, "it *isn't* personal." Awareness of this point helps the expert to avoid unduly defensive reactions that tend to undermine witness credibility.

Moreover, certain personal questions might arguably *become* relevant insofar as they demonstrate an actual or potential bias in relation to the case or to the underlying issue being litigated. But separating the intrusive, provocative chaff from the potentially relevant wheat is often difficult, especially on the witness stand, and little guidance is available for the witness in that situation. Some scholars suggest that the more clinical/experiential (versus research-based) the basis for the expert's opinion, the more compelling the arguments that personal information about the expert may be relevant to that opinion. However, the matter can hardly be considered settled by that point alone.

Experts surely vary in how they respond to personal and intrusive questions in the heat of trial, and an expert might legitimately feel that a particular query was simply too personal to be answered on the stand. But no data currently exist showing how experts determine to their own satisfaction whether a potentially relevant personal question crosses the line into inappropriateness. The pilot study described below explored this question (2).

Pilot Study

Method

Members of the Program in Psychiatry and the Law at the Harvard Medical School and attendees at a workshop on attorney-expert relations held at the 1999 annual meeting of the American Academy of Psychiatry and the Law completed questionnaires that asked subjects to rate the appropriateness of a series of personal questions asked of experts in contexts that might possibly justify their relevance. Presumably, the majority of respondents were forensically sophisticated and experienced in providing testimony. Responses on 37 usable questionnaires were rated on a scale from 1 (appropriate) to 6 (too personal, and hence inappropriate). Subjects were asked to explain their responses. Responses were measured against the indifference point of 3.5 (see [2]). Results were analyzed and are presented below.

Results

1. (Custody case) "Doctor, have you been divorced?"
   No significant trend emerged, but there was a modal peak at "too personal" (35%) and a remarkably flat distribution across all other responses (mean=2.94, SD=1.89).

   Sample comments:

   Subject #17: Mildly intrusive.

   Subject #27: This may be fair—if not used as a diversion, but better to avoid.

   Subject #31: Personal, but public record anyway.

   Subject #35: Might go to possible unconscious bias.

2. "What were the circumstances of the [expert's own] divorce?"(who divorced whom, stated or actual grounds, etc.)
   Here, in contrast to the last query, respondents gave the strongest response of the survey: a statistically significant response (76%) of "too personal" (mean=1.42, SD=1.02, $P<0.0001$).

   Sample comments:

   Subject #14: Extremely personal—beyond the pale—could not possibly be relevant and simply serves to embarrass the expert.

Subject #15: Too nosy—unrelated to my opinions.

Subject #36: Although some logic may apply as in above questions, believe [it] is inappropriate (although I'm not logically following through).

3. "Doctor, have you had any substance abuse problems?"
Here a statistically significant finding (65%) of "too personal" was the result—the second-clearest trend in the survey (mean=2.00, SD=1.77, $P<0.0001$).

Sample comments:

Subject #15: My medical history is not a credential.

Subject #21: Cannot envisage relevancy except to get emotional response from me.

Subject #29: I strongly believe there are no reasons for personal questions.

4. (Emotional injury case) "Doctor, what percentage of your income derives from forensic work?"
This fairly common query produced the only result that showed a significant bias toward "appropriate" (mean=4.49, SD=1.22, $P<0.0001$).

Sample comments:

Subject #2: I believe it is reasonable to ask what percentage of my work is forensic, and I always answer questions about how much I'm earning on the case at hand. I would have trouble getting closer to a discussion about actual income.

Subject #15: This doesn't bother me as it reflects my activities and CV [curriculum vitae].

Subject #26: I think one needs to answer percentage of work (NOT INCOME) from forensics—50:50 leans against hired gun.

Subject #30: Believe with specialty of forensic psychiatry, this is no longer synonymous with hired gun, so basically irrelevant. No difference.

5. (Same case as previous question) "Doctor, what is your income?"
This query showed a modal peak of "too personal" (62.2%), but not to the point of statistical significance (mean=1.60, SD=0.98, $P<0.0001$).

Sample comments:

Subject #5: Only IRS should know.

Subject #14: Could not be relevant to case. Jury assumes all doctors make a lot of money (wrong!).

Subject #17: How is this relevant? Damaging only.

Subject #34: I have not ever had this question allowed by the judge; inappropriate.

6. (Testamentary capacity case) "Doctor, do you have a will?" (moving party = disgruntled heirs)
    No clear position emerged on this point, with results paralleling chance distribution. There was a nonsignificant trend toward "too personal."

    Sample comments:

    Subject #15: Too subjective, though not offensively personal.

    Subject #17: This is mildly intrusive but not overly personal.

    Subject #21: It may have some relevancy.

7. (Malpractice case in which an alcoholic man committed suicide) "Doctor, are you an alcoholic?"
    Here again there was a nonsignificant trend toward "too personal" but no consensus (mean=2.89, SD=1.51, $P<0.02$).

    Sample comments:

    Subject #5: Just feels too personal.

    Subject #27: Might be helpful if conveyed with empathy.

    Subject #35: Irrelevant and inflammatory.

8. (Expert has been retained to do an insanity evaluation of a spree killer who has sworn to kill homosexuals and has killed several persons thought by him to be homosexual) "Doctor, are you homosexual?"
    While no significant trend emerged, a nearly significant trend toward "too personal" was revealed; that was also the modal answer (mean=2.14, SD=1.67, $P<0.0001$).

Sample comments:

Subject #10: What happens in bed is my business.

Subject #15: This would tend to be prejudicial, and I would expect that a judge would bar it.

Subject #27: If I were homosexual I would feel different—*maybe*.

9. (Expert has been retained to evaluate an ex–altar boy for emotional harms from sexual abuse by Catholic priest): "Doctor, are you Catholic?"

    This query elicited a chance distribution, but a nonsignificant majority believed this question to be fair game (mean=3.2, SD=1.73).

    Sample comments:

    Subject #12: Relevant if you want to be a Supreme Judicial Court justice in Massachusetts.

    Subject #15: Personal, but not top secret. I would be reluctant.

    Subject #17: This may be relevant to formulation of the case and is only mildly intrusive.

    Subject #26: Attorney may wish to know if expert is familiar with Catholic church system—does veer toward personal.

Discussion

As the study results indicate, little consensus could be derived from responses to a variety of personal queries with varying relevance to the forensic matter at hand. Respondents did feel strongly that inquiry about the circumstances of the expert's divorce were clearly too personal and thus inappropriate, though queries about the *fact* of the divorce showed little agreement. Respondents also accepted the appropriateness of a question about what percentage of the expert's income derived from forensic work but felt (nonsignificantly) that a query as to the actual income was too personal.

Little guidance is offered to the expert faced with such questions in a deposition or trial, and relatively few resources address this issue directly. In recent work Babitsky and Mangraviti devote several pages to this issue (3, 4). These authors make this point:

Remember that as a witness in a case your credibility is a major issue. Thus, questions about licensing, criminal convictions, fees earned, suspensions, exclusion of prior testimony, prior expert witnessing work, etc. are all fair game and should be answered without hesitation. (3, pp. 224–225)

The authors note that the test of the appropriateness of personal questions is "reasonableness." Federal Rule of Evidence 611 gives a judge authority to exercise control over questioning "to protect the witnesses from harassment or undue embarrassment" (5). According to 7 Federal Procedure, "The deponent has no redress unless the annoyance, embarrassment or oppression will be unreasonable, and the seeking of information is not unreasonably annoying, embarrassing or oppressive if the information is material and relevant" (6, p. 654).

If an expert witness is accompanied to a deposition by his or her personal attorney, the latter may instruct the expert not to answer a given question, but the retaining attorney usually may not. At controversial junctures, depositions can be suspended and the matter argued out before a judge. An expert may seek a protective order from the judge permitting him or her not to answer a question.

The following answer would probably be safe but open to judicial challenge upon the proper motion by the questioning attorney: "I choose not to answer that question as it is too personal, but I will attest that my (marital status, income, substance abuse history if any, etc.) does not affect my opinion in this case." Case law varies considerably on the issue of divulging personal income. Although some jurisdictions provide some form of protection regarding this disclosure, others (e.g., Maryland) require that an expert who derives "substantial" income from forensic practice disclose the amount. A recent case contains a review of case law on this point (7).

In an actual trial, however, the expert is largely at the whim of the judge's rulings on personal questions, since—unlike in deposition—one's personal attorney does not attend. While most judges are reasonable about such matters, an occasional jurist may be too passive, curious, or impaired to bar the expert's answer. The expert must then face the highly stressful prospect of refusing to answer and risking contempt of court, or answering the query and experiencing the consequent exposure, which is now a matter of public record and may well reside on mainframe computers indefinitely. The only useful advice that can be given to the expert at this juncture is to pick one's battles, that is, to reserve outright refusal for the most serious, least forensically relevant queries.

References

1. Brodsky SL: The Expert Expert Witness: More Maxims and Guidelines for Testifying in Court. Washington, DC, American Psychological Association, 1999
2. Gutheil TG, Commons ML, Miller PM: Personal questions on cross-examination: a pilot study of expert witness attitudes. J Am Acad Psychiatry Law 29:85–88, 2001
3. Babitsky S, Mangraviti JJ: How to Excel During Depositions: Techniques for Experts That Work. Falmouth, MA, SEAK, Inc., 1999
4. Babitsky S, Mangraviti JJ: How to Excel During Cross-Examination: Techniques for Experts That Work. Falmouth, MA, SEAK, Inc., 1997
5. Federal Rules of Evidence, Rule 611: Mode and order of interrogation and presentation
6. Federal Procedure, Lawyer's Edition. Rochester, NY, Lawyers Co-operative Publishing Company, 1994, p 654
7. Wrobleski v DeLara, 121 Md App 181, 708 A. 2d 1086 (1998)

9

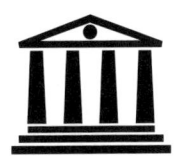

Telling Tales Out of Court

Experts' Disclosures About Opposing Experts

> It is unethical for a physician to disparage the professional competence, knowledge, qualifications or services of another physician to a patient or a third party.
>
> American College of Physicians (1)

A number of sources, including, by implication, the Supreme Court case *Ake v. Oklahoma*, have stated or implied that consultation provided to the retaining attorney by the expert witness is a legitimate expert function (2–6). Indeed, it is extremely common for one

---

This chapter was adapted from Gutheil TG, Commons ML, Miller PM: "'Telling Tales Out of Court': A Pilot Study of Experts' Disclosures About Opposing Experts." *Journal of the American Academy of Psychiatry and the Law* 28:449–453, 2000. Used with permission.

side's expert to offer the retaining attorney consultative assistance by pointing out weaknesses, mistaken assumptions, flawed clinical reasoning, and unsupported conclusions in the other expert's opinion. Such consultation is intended to aid the attorney in critiquing the opposing expert's report, preparing for the opposing expert's deposition, and (if a case reaches trial) in designing cross-examination of the opposing expert.

Regardless of whether *Ake v. Oklahoma* is explicitly considered, experts and attorneys generally accept, and even expect, such consultative participation by the expert; the legitimacy of this function is rarely questioned. The caveat that such consultation steers dangerously close to advocacy for the *case*, rather than for one's opinion (2), is readily answered by noting that the expert merely extends the traditional educational role intrinsic to all expert witness functioning (first educating the attorney, then the fact finder) by continuing to educate the attorney about psychiatric theory, knowledge, and reasoning—but, in this instance, about those elements in the opinion of the opposing expert.

Beyond these familiar, case-centered functions, however, there exists a gray zone of information that experts might or might not choose to disclose to their retaining attorneys. This information might include relevant issues of credentialing—such as whether the other expert is board certified, widely respected, published in the area under consideration, a member of the AAPL (American Academy of Psychiatry and the Law)—and similar, largely public information. Such data are fairly readily available from the other expert's curriculum vitae, directories and other organizational information sources, literature searches, and, currently, even on the Internet. Other information of a more personal nature might well be known to members of the relatively small forensic, academic, or regional community, but certain constraints—be they considerations of ethics, personal values, good manners, or even good taste—might lead an expert to decline to share all that he or she knows with the attorney. Indeed, the expert may feel the tension of walking the line between legitimate expert consultative functions and what amounts to slander of a peer.

What Is Personal Information?

Within the court context there are two broad types of limitations on informational disclosure: 1) relevance to the case matter at hand and 2) rules, statutes, and constitutional provisions that address privacy. To work within the legal system is to accept that ultimately the courts, not the expert, decide what is relevant and privileged. But much of our current subject lies outside the procedure-driven world of the courtroom; most such disclosures, if they occur, emerge in private conversations between attorney and expert.

Addressing a subject that has rarely been systematically explored, this chapter describes some preliminary empirical work that polled practitioners about what kinds of information about opposing experts is and is not considered proper to disclose. We begin by attempting to divide our subject matter into categories.

Information about a person may be divided into three realms of discourse: 1) private (information relating to one's personal life and shared only in confidence), 2) social (information one might share with acquaintances at a party), and 3) public (information generally available through resumes, court records, lectures, publications, and the like). We propose that the soundest ethical position for the expert witness is to apply the ethical constraint of protecting the private and social realms of discourse, including disclosures about opposing experts, from exposure to one's retaining attorney.

Pilot Study

The diverse content that characterizes the informational gray zone of expert-expert disclosure is commonly discussed at any gathering where forensic practitioners have the opportunity to analyze or complain about the opinions, testimony, or behavior of colleagues, and to gossip, dish, and share rumors about the public and personal lives of fellow practitioners. Though this behavior is perhaps common to all social gatherings, discussion in the literature of its relevance to formal expert witness practice is extremely scanty (6); neither the content nor the decision-making process involved in such disclosures has ever been studied systematically. The pilot study performed by the Program in Psychiatry and the Law at the Massachusetts Mental Health Center and reported in this chapter attempts to address this omission in order to learn how experts actually regard various forms of disclosure under differing circumstances and how they view professionalism, and to gain added insight into how they function (7).

The study began with the hypothesis that some disclosures would be generally acceptable, particularly in the realm of public data, and that other, more personal data, particularly of a stigmatizing nature, might well be withheld. Beyond this sharp public/private distinction, the study sought to determine from the sample polled whether there might be subgroups within the expert witness community that would tend toward marked reticence about a fellow expert in any area other than the latter's expressed opinion. The study also examined whether there might be other subgroups that would be less constrained, based on the philosophy that all data, no matter how obtained, how relevant, or how derogatory, are fair game for the adversary system and may be shared under the general expert mandate.

Method

Participant Description

The participant sample consisted of 1) those members of the Program in Psychiatry and the Law who had played no role in designing the questionnaire and 2) attendees at a workshop entitled "Attorney-Expert Twilight Zone," advertised as focusing on unexplored aspects of expert witness practice. The latter workshop was held at the 1999 annual meeting of the AAPL. The study hypothesis assumed that subjects (mostly AAPL members) were interested in forensic practice and varied in their levels of experience. Clearly neither representative nor random, the sample was chosen according to the following logic: the title of the seminar might be presumed to attract those interested in the topic who could readily express opinions on "right behavior," regardless of their actual experience with the situations described in the proffered questionnaire.

Questionnaire Design

Participants filled out questionnaires that inquired about a variety of issues, including a spectrum of possible disclosures—ranging from those that might be considered objective and factual to those that would be considered highly subjective and personal—that one side's expert might or might not make to the retaining attorney about the opposing expert. Participants were asked to imagine what behavior would be appropriate for an expert witness, even if they had never faced a particular situation in practice.

Questions were organized in order of increasing encroachment on personal privacy or increasing possible stigma from the information to be disclosed. In some cases the nature of the legal case in question was given to imply the possible relevance of the disclosure in identifying a potential source of bias. Respondents were asked to rate whether the disclosure was ethical or appropriate on a 10-point scale, where 1 equaled "never appropriate" and 10 signified "always appropriate." A score of 5.5 indicated the statistical indifference point. Thus, the numerical responses were tested as they differed significantly from 5.5.

In each instance a follow-up query asked, on a similar 10-point scale, how relevant disclosure of that issue was to the function of an expert witness in the situation described.

Note that 1) this was a limited pilot study and 2) a small percentage of the questionnaires were completed by members of the Program who had not participated in designing the questionnaires.

Results

A total of 37 usable questionnaires were returned for analysis, a response rate of approximately one-third. Many contained one or more elements of missing data. Even with the missing data, the following conclusions could be supported by the evidence: 1) disclosure of the publicly available factual material was regarded as fully acceptable by large majorities and 2) the more personal data evoked significant scatter in the responses. Some questions identified subgroups of respondents who supported either "Yes" or "No" responses. The questions and the responses are summarized as follows: frequency distributions, means, and standard deviations of responses and results of t tests are provided, as well as a principal component analysis limited to two factors. For all the t tests, the means obtained are compared to a chance rating of 5.5—halfway between totally inappropriate (1) and totally appropriate (10).

The following five queries may be considered to constitute the "public" data on the opposing expert—data based mostly on information theoretically available from a curriculum vitae or court records. Responses with respect to appropriateness of such disclosure were uniform. Participants also found questions 3, 4, and 5 (but not 1 and 2) relevant to the function of an expert witness.

1. "The other expert is not board certified."

    When compared to a chance rating of 5.5, the mean rating of 8.7 on this item suggests that participants found this disclosure appropriate (mean=8.7, SD=2.0, $t(36)=9.8$, $P=0.000$).

2. "The other expert is not *forensic* board certified."

    Results here were almost identical to those for the first question (mean=8.1, SD=2.3, $t(36)=6.7$, $P=0.000$). Separate investigations confirmed that subjects likely grasped the two concepts being queried—that is, they understood "board certified" to indicate "certified in general psychiatry" and "forensic board certified" to mean "certified in forensic psychiatry by either the American Board (the original forensic board) or having added qualifications in forensic psychiatry (the 'new board' category of the ABPN)."

3. "The other expert does cases only for one side (plaintiff/prosecution/defense)."

   Respondents accepted this disclosure at a level significantly above chance (mean=8.4, SD=2.2, $t(36)=7.9$, $P=0.000$). There was a nonsignificant trend toward the view that this disclosure *was* relevant to expert function.

4. "The other expert's lecture last year on this very subject reveals a bias."

   Results were broadly comparable to those in Question 3 above (mean=8.4, SD=2.0, $t(36)=8.8$, $P=0.000$).

5. "The other expert's recent article on subject matter related to this case reveals a bias."

   Again, results paralleled Question 3 above (mean=8.6, SD=1.7, $t(36)=10.7$, $P=0.000$).

Results were quite different with the more personal queries as follows. Instead of responding that the queries were "appropriate" as happened for the most part with the first five questions, subjects most frequently indicated "inappropriate" to the following seven questions.

1. "The other expert is a survivor of childhood sexual abuse and probably cannot be objective about this recovered memory case."

   Responses here were scattered, with a large standard deviation (mean=4.0, SD=3.2, $t(36)=-3.0$, $P=0.005$). Interestingly, there was a plurality in favor of "never appropriate," yet nine respondents indicated it was almost always acceptable to disclose this.

2. "The other expert has been through a messy divorce and custody battle and is thus questionably objective about this custody case."

   Amid scattered responses with a large standard deviation (mean=4.2, SD=3.4, $t(36)=-2.3$, $P=0.029$), the modal answer, with a slight statistical significance, was "never appropriate."

3. "The other expert is gay/lesbian and thus is questionably objective in this emotional injury case involving gay bashing."

   Responses against disclosure were significant, with the mode at "never appropriate" (mean=3.8, SD=3.2, $t(36)=-3.2$, $p=.003$).

4. "The other expert is known to me personally to be an alcoholic" (in a case involving alcoholism).

   The modal answer was "never appropriate" (mean=3.8, SD=3.1, $t(36)=-3.2$, $P=0.003$).

5. "The other expert is known to me personally to be a substance abuser" (in a case involving substance abuse).

    Participants favored *not* disclosing this (mode=2) even though responses showed some scatter (mean=3.7, SD=3.0, $t(36)=-3.6$, $P=0.001$).

6. "The other expert is known to me personally to be a liar."

    Again, participants favored nondisclosure (mode=2) even though responses showed some scatter (mean=4.1, SD=3.0, $t(36)=-2.7$, $P=0.010$).

7. "The other expert is known to me personally to be a member of a hate group (KKK, survivalist militia, skinhead group, etc.)."

    Surprisingly, the responses to this query revealed a statistically significant finding *toward* appropriateness of disclosure (mean=7.1, SD=3.1, $t(36)=3.1$, $P=0.004$), accompanied by a similar agreement that this disclosure *was* relevant to expert witness function (mean=7.6, SD=2.5, $t(36)=4.8$, $P=0.000$). Though comparably personal when compared to (and perhaps more stigmatizing than) earlier hypothetical disclosures, this query identifies a semipublic role (i.e., political group membership), which may explain why this query yielded a different response.

In most of the last seven questions above, responses regarding the second dimension, "relevance to expert witness function," were widely scattered and hence inconclusive. The exception was Question 12, about being a member of a hate group.

Factor analysis of the data revealed two major factors. The variables that load on each factor support grouping the questions into two main constructs: 1) the publicly available data, which are generally viewed as suitable for disclosure and 2) a set of "personal secrets," for whom the appropriateness of disclosure evoked wide variability of opinion among respondents to this survey, with a trend toward keeping the secret.

Discussion

Since only a pilot study is described, it is clear that further investigations must involve larger numbers of participants with a wider range of backgrounds. The study data are also limited to what respondents *say* they would do, or what they say should appropriately be done, rather than what they *actually* do "behind closed doors."

A relatively clear distinction between disclosure of private and public data did emerge. However, beyond the simple public/private distinction we may find it noteworthy—and, perhaps, even somewhat distressing—that for "personal" data, responses were so widely scattered, indicating that there is little consensus or agreement about the suitability of personal disclosures. This is the case despite the fact that many of the personal data used in the questionnaire would be the kind of information highly subject to rumor, hearsay, thirdhand information, innuendo, personal bias or animus in the reporter, and similar distorting influences. An example might be Question 7, in relation to which an expert would be unlikely to know all of the facts about an opposing expert's difficult divorce case. These findings about the willingness of some experts to consider revealing personal information clearly suggest a need to discuss these issues in open fora with the possible goal of at least some movement toward consensus in such critical matters.

These results reveal interesting parallels with two earlier studies in other realms: one on mental health professionals' attitudes toward sex between patients (8) and a second on the imagined duty of therapists to report patients' past crimes (9). Both those studies and the present one capture the notion of "professional duties," a notion characteristic of the systematic reasoning stage of moral development (10).

At this developmental stage a person's roles within a system are seen as public. All such roles have a public dimension in contrast to their private aspect, but unlike some of them, professional work in the real world is usually open to examination and critique. Forensic psychiatrists, for example, must testify clearly in open court and clarify the basis of each opinion so that lay juries can understand both the opinion and the reasoning behind it. The forensic context is a public one, occurring in open court, with essentially permanent stenographic recording; fittingly, the disclosures in our survey that addressed public data were seen to be appropriate.

The information disclosed in the public realm was distinguished from that which might be appropriately considered secret. The personal information known to the expert was separate from the expert's public (professional) role. This position contrasts markedly with more primitive conceptual models in which the private person and the (public) role are inappropriately joined (or confused) in the observer's eye (10).

Ethical Issues

Although our study was primarily aimed at determining what our sample thought would be appropriate disclosure by one expert about another expert in specific situations, both the issue and the responses raise certain larger ethical questions. Our general position is that the minimal acceptable requirement for an expert is to maintain professional standards, which would include 1) avoiding conflicts of interest, 2) refraining from disclosing private material about either clients, patients, *or* the other expert, and 3) maintaining professional judgment despite various pressures deriving either directly from attorneys or from the stresses of testifying under oath.

The ethics code of the American Academy of Psychiatry and the Law identifies fairly clearly the expert's duties to examinees but offers little explicit guidance on dealing either with attorneys or opposing experts. In general terms, the criterion of honesty and striving for objectivity includes the idea that the expert's opinion "reflects this honesty and efforts to attain objectivity" (Appendix 11–1, Guideline IV). The commentary on Guideline IV of the ethics code specifically says the following:

> Practicing forensic psychiatrists enhance the honesty and objectivity of their work by basing their forensic opinions, forensic reports, and forensic testimony on *all the data available to them*. They communicate the honesty of their work, efforts to attain objectivity, and the soundness of their clinical opinion by *distinguishing to the extent possible between verified and unverified information*, as well as among clinical 'facts,' 'inferences,' and 'impressions.'[emphases added] (Appendix 11–1, Guideline IV)

Based on the foregoing, one could justify *not* providing one's retaining lawyer with information about the other side's expert because of the difficulty in discriminating between "verified and unverified information," but that question is obviated if, in fact, the information is directly and validly known to the expert. On the other hand, a case could be made that the principles of honesty and striving for objectivity at a minimum permit the expert to tell the attorney candidly what one expert knows about the other. Further, objectivity would theoretically be served because certain kinds of knowledge about the opposing expert could help identify a potential bias that might ultimately be illuminating to the jury if exposed during cross-examination. Both of these latter rationales may be seen to derive from the phrase "all the data available" in the ethics commentary. Although it is actually more likely that the framers of this code had in mind the *clinical* data relating to the examinee or to the forensic issue at stake, the decision to disclose could thus be defended in relation to material such as that presented in the study described above. Professionals, however, understand not only the stated, literal portions of ethical codes but also the reasons for statement of those principles and their implications for situations not explicitly described (see, for example, [11], which notes that ethics codes offer only minimal guidance but should provide basic principles to guide decision making). A more fundamental argument could be made that critique of an opposing expert's *opinion* legitimately uses those clinical skills for which one has been retained, while disclosure of more personal information lies outside that realm of legitimacy. Appelbaum has put this with characteristic clarity:

> Information about a witness's private life ("He's going through a divorce and might be a little shaky now") or professional reputation unrelated to the opinion being offered in the current case ("I understand he's a hired gun for sale to the highest bidder") does not serve to advance the interests of ascertaining truth in the courtroom. An aggressive attorney might well like to know such information and might find it of use in attacking an opposing witness, but it should not be the role of the forensic expert to provide it. (6, p. 24)

Appelbaum's decisive answer—with which we are in full agreement—contrasts markedly with the wide scatter of responses on our survey, a contrast that forcefully suggests that the issue requires further discussion.

Unaddressed in our study is the personal ethical self-scrutiny that might, for example, lead an expert to avoid taking on a custody case in the middle of, or shortly after, a messy divorce situation. In that sense, the expert attempts to maximize striving for objectivity by taking affirmative steps to avoid potential personal bias.

We further suggest that an *impression* formed about an opposing expert ("I think that expert only takes cases for the defense"), if conveyed as if it were a known fact, represents a failure of the ethics of objectivity. While *objectivity*, as used in the ethics guidelines, may focus primarily on the posture of the expert toward the examinee or the clinical question at issue, the requirement for objectivity could easily be understood (and appropriately so) to extend to the opposing expert as well. Undocumented hearsay cannot be considered the kind of objective data about which the expert should be educating the attorney.

Conclusion

In conclusion, the survey results presented above imply that respondents for the most part viewed their expert functions and those of the opposing expert as public and open. In choosing what to disclose, respondents operated more from their professional and scientific roles than from the role of someone privy to the personal secrets and presumed biases of the opposing expert. Insofar as these responses mirror actual practice, the findings are generally encouraging as to the professionalism and judgment of respondents. The wide scatter on some responses, however, clearly indicates the need for both open discussion about, and further study of, these issues.

References

1. Position paper, Ethics Manual, 4th Edition, American College of Physicians. Ann Intern Med 128:576–594, 1998
2. Gutheil TG: The Psychiatrist as Expert Witness. Washington, DC, American Psychiatric Press, 1998
3. Appelbaum PS, Gutheil TG: Clinical Handbook of Psychiatry and the Law, 3rd Edition. Baltimore, MD, Williams & Wilkins, 2000
4. Berger SH: Establishing a Forensic Psychiatric Practice. New York, WW Norton, 1997
5. Ake v Oklahoma, 105 S Ct 1087, (1985)
6. Appelbaum PS: In the wake of *Ake*: the ethics of expert testimony in an advocate's world. Bull Am Acad Psychiatry Law 15:15–25, 1987
7. Gutheil TG, Commons ML, Miller PM: "Telling tales out of court": a pilot study of experts' disclosures about opposing experts. J Am Acad Psychiatry Law 28:449–453, 2000
8. Commons ML, Bohn JT, Godon LM, et al: Professionals' attitudes towards sex between institutionalized patients. Am J Psychother 46:571–580, 1992
9. Commons ML, Lee P, Gutheil TG, et al: Moral stage of reasoning and the misperceived "duty" to report past crimes (misprision). Int J Law Psychiatry 18:415–424, 1995
10. Colby A, Kohlberg L: The Measurement of Moral Judgment, Vol 1: Theoretical Foundations and Research Validation. New York, Cambridge University Press, 1987
11. Handselman MM: Confidentiality: the ethical baby in the legal bath water. J Applied Rehab Counseling 18:33–34, 1989

10

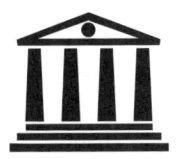

Effects of the *Daubert* Case on Preparing Psychiatric/Psychological Testimony for Court

Scholars from a number of fields have expressed concern for many years about the introduction of so-called "junk science" into the courtroom (1). Moreover, when expert testimony proved decisive but was suspect, overturning a lower court decision on admissibility of expert evidence was subject to the standard of abuse of discretion. That is, to overturn a lower court decision, an appellate court was required to conclude that the trial court had committed an error of law. Under this standard, it is difficult to overturn a judge's decision to admit or exclude an expert's testimony.

This chapter was adapted from Gutheil TG, Stein M: "*Daubert*-Based Gatekeeping and Psychiatric/Psychological Testimony in Court: Review and Proposal." *Journal of Psychiatry and the Law* 28:235–251, 2000. Used with permission.

Concerns about increased acceptance of questionable expertise in court were eased, if not laid to rest, in a series of Supreme Court cases, particularly the opinion in *Kumho Tire,* with its strong reaffirmation of a trial court's "gatekeeper" role in screening, and sometimes excluding, doubtful expert assessments (2). The gatekeeper role creates its own problems, however: trial courts are obligated to make initial determinations about whether a jury can consider the views of one or more experts in areas in which a judge is not likely to have much experience or specialized training. Fortunately, the justices of the Supreme Court have provided guidance as to how a trial judge should carry out such gate keeping.

As articulated by the Court, a trial judge is to perform the gatekeeping function "to make certain that an expert, *whether basing testimony upon professional studies or personal experience,* employs in the courtroom the same level of intellectual rigor that characterizes the practice of an expert in the relevant field" [emphasis added] (2, p. 1176). The underlined phrase may have particular relevance to psychiatric or psychological testimony since clinical experience counts so heavily in those fields.

This chapter explores the details of how mental health professionals can assist the courts in carrying out their responsibilities in light of proven techniques used by psychiatrists and psychologists that would fall within the guidelines provided by the case law above and the Federal Rules of Evidence.

Daubert, Joiner, and *Kumho*: The Expert Witness Trilogy

The *Daubert* Case

The important Supreme Court case *Daubert v. Merrell Dow Pharmaceuticals* proposed a benchmark for admissibility of expert witness testimony based, in a highly condensed summary, on whether that testimony is relevant and reliable and will help the fact finder to understand a point at issue (3; the case is reviewed in detail elsewhere [4]). Though applicable only to federal courts, the ramifications of *Daubert* have led other jurisdictions to follow the standards set in this case and in a series of subsequent ones, often referred to as "*Daubert* progeny," that further elaborate the basic points of the case (2, 5). These decisions have far-reaching implications for expert witnesses, litigating parties, and clinical research.

Even where local case law has not yet adopted this standard, the wise expert notwithstanding applies these criteria of relevance to the case at hand to forestall a *Daubert*-based challenge to the admissibility of the proffered opinion—a challenge that might exclude it from admission entirely. That is, the expert scrutinizes his or her opinion to check 1) its relevance to the case at hand, 2) the scientific reliability of the reasoning and conclusion, and 3) its utility in aiding the fact finder to understand the point at issue.

In *Daubert* the Supreme Court set itself the task of determining "the standard for admitting expert scientific testimony in a federal trial" under the Federal Rules of Evidence (3, p. 582). The Federal Rules of Evidence went into effect in 1973. Fifty years earlier the then Court of Appeals for the District of Columbia had articulated the "general acceptance" test for the admission of an expert's testimony at trial, namely, that "while courts will go a long way in admitting expert testimony deduced from a well-recognized scientific principle or discovery, *the thing from which the deduction is made must be sufficiently established to have gained general acceptance in the particular field in which it belongs*" (6, quoted in 3, p. 586 [emphasis added by the Supreme Court]).

In *Daubert*, the lower courts had excluded the plaintiff's medical experts from testifying, and judgment had entered for Merrell Dow. The legal analysis supporting these actions was that Daubert's experts had based their conclusions on methods not generally accepted in the medical research field. The Supreme Court ruled that the *Frye* test had been superseded: "*Frye* made 'general acceptance' the exclusive test for admitting expert testimony. That austere standard, absent from, and incompatible with, the Federal Rules of Evidence, should not be applied in federal trials" (3, p.589).

The Supreme Court reasoned that not only was there no consideration of *Frye* in the legislative history, but that "a rigid 'general acceptance' requirement would be at odds with the 'liberal thrust' of the Federal Rules and their 'general approach of relaxing the traditional barriers to "opinion" testimony'" (3, quoting from 7 and citing Rules 701–705). The Court went on to balance the "open door" the Federal Rules of Evidence provided for admitting expert testimony against the countervailing consideration that "the trial judge must ensure that any and all scientific testimony or evidence admitted is not only relevant, but *reliable*" (3, p. 589). Finally, the opinion made clear that its discussion, which arose in a case discussing hard medical research, was confined to scientific expertise under Federal Rule of Evidence 702.

The Court went on to list some factors that could be considered to establish scientific reliability, for example, testing, peer review and publication, and known or potential rate of error (3, pp. 593–594). In this discussion, general acceptance can be considered, but only as one factor:

Widespread acceptance can be an important factor in ruling particular evidence admissible, and "a known technique which has been able to attract only minimal support within the community" (*[United States v.] Downing*, 753 F. 2d. at 1238) may properly be viewed with skepticism. (3, p. 594)

Daubert answered *some* questions about the standards for admitting expert testimony but left open many others that were significant. One was whether its discussion of some factors for determining reliability of "hard" scientific evidence was equally applicable to "soft" expertise based on "other specialized knowledge," such as the clinical experience of psychiatrists, psychologists, and social workers. Many courts concluded that it did not. This created the possibility of a so-called expert assuring a court that his or her analysis was well founded even if not grounded in any objectively established methodology. When a jury has been presented with testimony by a so-called expert, and that testimony has been admitted, it becomes a basis for a jury decision that is very difficult to reverse.

Example

In a sexual harassment lawsuit, the plaintiff's expert psychiatrist concluded that the plaintiff had suffered psychological harm as a result of the conduct of her supervisor. The sole basis for this assessment was the version of events provided by the plaintiff. There were contradictory narratives available in the database (records) from the defendant and from neutral witnesses, for example, 1) a conversation with the supervisor that the plaintiff saw as intimidating, while a co-worker who was present saw no such content and 2) the plaintiff's refusal to give up a computer password lest material be retrieved to be used against her. Moreover, the plaintiff espoused actual conspiracy theories about her supervisor, her co-workers, and others.

Faced with such data, a forensic evaluator would be required by the standard of care for expert practice to consider and attempt to rule out clinical disorders such as histrionic personality disorder, borderline personality disorder, or one of the paranoid conditions, all of which are well recognized in the literature as causing difficulties with the accurate interpretation of human interactions while yet permitting a person to function adequately in an office setting. These disorders have long been recognized as contributing to a subjective perception of sexual harassment even in its absence (8). For these reasons, the competent expert faced with these data is obligated to rule out the possible impact of these conditions, since they are not causally related to workplace factors.

The expert retained by the plaintiff's attorney in the above example performed an inadequate forensic assessment. First, basic forensic methodology requires considering readily available collateral sources of information, especially discorroborating ones. Second, the expert could readily have employed psychological testing, the most efficient, reliable, and solidly validated method of addressing such questions. A standard battery of psychological tests, relied on for decades by both clinicians and forensic evaluators, presents reliable and objective data than can be used to address the questions noted above. These tests are the most thoroughly researched and well-established measures of mental functioning in modern psychology and psychiatry. They reveal attempts at feigning, minimizing, or exaggerating mental conditions (9). Without such examination of collateral sources and/or testing, the evaluation by the plaintiff's psychiatrist—which relied exclusively on the plaintiff's interpretation of the intentions and meanings of communications by those around her—was inadequate and incomplete.

Note for clarity that this example is not proffered to suggest that psychological testing is mandatory in all forensic evaluations. Indeed, careful forensic examination of the litigant coupled with thorough exhaustion of collateral data may provide a sufficient basis for valid and reliable forensic psychiatric conclusions to be drawn.

Note further that when psychological testing *is* employed, the psychiatrist-expert should generally not testify as to the reliability or validity of the instruments themselves unless he or she has had specific training in that subject; the examining psychologist may clearly offer such reliability/validity data and should be prepared to do so.

Under the standard eventually adopted by the Supreme Court in *Kumho Tire* (2, see discussion below), the testimony of the plaintiff's psychiatrist in the case described above might well have been excluded on methodological grounds. His failure to consider collateral sources or administer the standard battery of psychological tests meant that he failed to "[employ] in the courtroom the same level of intellectual rigor that characterizes the practice of an expert in the relevant field" (2, p. 1176). Instead of having psychological tests administered to his client, the plaintiff's attorney actually went to court and obtained an order from the trial judge that such tests were *not* to be administered!

The *Joiner* Case

Returning to the development of case law regarding the admissibility of expert evidence, we come to the next Supreme Court case in the "forensic expert trilogy": *General Electric Co. v. Joiner* (5). The issue in that case was whether Joiner's exposure to certain chemicals caused Joiner's lung cancer. The trial judge excluded the testimony offered by Joiner's experts, concluding that it "did not rise above 'subjective belief or unsupported speculation'" (5, p. 516). The appellate court held the position that with regard to expert testimony, the Federal Rules of Evidence "display a preference for admissibility," and, applying a stricter standard of review to the trial court's exclusion of a forensic expert, it reversed the previous ruling. This reasoning is exactly what many feared would follow from *Daubert*, opening a Pandora's box and freeing a host of "experts" upon the courts whose methodologies and speculations would be looked upon with skepticism by their professional colleagues.

The Supreme Court reversed the appellate court's decision, reinstating the trial judge's exclusion of the proposed experts. The legal basis for its action was that the decision to exclude was to be reviewed under the usual standard: did the judge abuse his or her discretion in making the ruling? In the analysis of why excluding the expert testimony did not exceed the judge's discretion, the Court announced that expertise does not exist in isolation:

> He [Joiner] claims that because the District Court's disagreement was with the conclusion that the experts drew from the studies, the District Court committed legal error and was properly reversed by the Court of Appeals. But conclusions and methodology are not entirely distinct from one another. Trained experts commonly extrapolate from existing data. But nothing in either *Daubert* or the Federal Rules of Evidence requires a district court to admit opinion evidence which is connected to existing data only by the ipse dixit of the expert. A court may conclude that there is simply too great an analytic gap between the data and the opinion proffered. . . . That is what the District Court did here, and we hold that it did not abuse its discretion in so doing. (5, p. 519) (citation omitted)

In a concurring opinion, Justice Breyer discussed a critical concern that the majority opinion did not choose to address, namely, if a judge has the responsibility to analyze whether the expert's opinion is supported by the data in a field in which the judge is not knowledgeable, and the judge cannot rely upon the expert's assurances of an analytic connection between the data and the opinion, how is this task to be carried out?

> Judges have increasingly found in the Rules of Evidence and Civil Procedure ways to help them overcome the inherent difficulty of making determinations about complicated scientific or otherwise technical evidence. Among these techniques are an increased use of Rule 16's [Fed

R. Civ. P], pretrial conference authority to narrow the scientific issues in dispute, pretrial hearings where potential experts are subject to examination by the court, and the appointment of special masters and specially trained law clerks. . . . In the present case, the New England Journal of Medicine has filed an amici brief . . . in which the Journal writes:

> A judge could better fulfill this gatekeeper function if he or she had help from scientists. Judges should be strongly encouraged to make greater use of their inherent authority . . . to appoint experts . . . Reputable experts could be recommended to courts by established scientific organizations, such as the National Academy of Sciences or the American Association for the Advancement of Science. . . . . cf. Fed. Rule Evid. 706 (court may "on its own motion or on the motion of any party" appoint an expert to serve on behalf of the court, and this expert may be selected as "agreed upon by the parties" or chosen by the court) . . . Given this kind of offer of cooperative effort, from the scientific to the legal community, and given the various Rules-authorized methods for facilitating the courts' task, it seems to me that *Daubert's* gate keeping requirement will not prove inordinately difficult to implement; and that it will help secure the basic objectives of the Federal Rules of Evidence; which are, to repeat, the ascertainment of truth and the just determination of proceedings. Fed. Rule Evid. 102. (5, pp. 520–521)

The *Kumho* Case

The last case in the expert witness trilogy is *Kumho Tire* (2). Whatever concerns *Daubert* may have raised about encouraging trial courts to favor the admission of expert testimony, and in the process lowering the threshold for "junk" expertise to be presented to juries, were laid to rest in *Kumho Tire*. This case arose out of a car accident caused by a tire blowing out. The question was whether the tire was defective, and the plaintiffs' case was primarily based on the testimony of a tire failure analyst. The trial court excluded his testimony and then entered judgment in favor of Kumho Tire, reasoning that several factors from *Daubert* "argued against the reliability of [the analyst's] methods" (2, p. 1173). On the initial appeal, the decision was reversed. The court of appeals concluded that the tire failure analyst based his conclusions on experience, rather than science, and therefore "'the district court erred as a matter of law by applying *Daubert* in this case'" (Id). When the Supreme Court took the matter up, it reversed the appeals court ruling:

> Nor, on the other hand, does the presence of *Daubert's* general acceptance factor help show that an expert's testimony is reliable where the discipline itself lacks reliability, as, for example, do theories grounded in any so-called generally accepted principles of astrology or necromancy.

> At the same time, ... some of *Daubert's* questions can help to evaluate the reliability even of experience-based testimony. In certain cases, it will be appropriate for the trial judge to ask ... whether such a method is generally accepted in the relevant ... community. Likewise, it will at times be useful to ask even of a witness whose expertise is based purely on experience ... whether his preparation is of a kind that others in the field would recognize as acceptable. (2, pp. 1175–1176)

This language answers several of the questions raised by *Daubert* and by lower court efforts to interpret the case. *Daubert* did not swing wide the gates to admit any testimony offered by a self-declared expert. Many of the factors it set out may be applicable to testimony grounded on experience, including acceptance of the methodology "in the relevant community." It is useful to recall that the author of the majority opinion in *Kumho Tire* is Justice Breyer, who wrote the concurring opinion in *Joiner*, which is discussed above. If read together they reveal a successful effort to raise with his Supreme Court colleagues the issue of ways in which a judge not trained in a particular discipline could avail himself or herself of resources in the relevant professional community in order to determine whether expert testimony is reliable (concurring opinion in *Joiner*). By the time *Kumho Tire* was decided a year and a half later, the Court as a whole took the next and most critical step and endorsed the idea that the legal standard for permitting expert testimony to be heard by the jury is the *very same standard* that the relevant professional community employs:

> The objective of ... [the *Daubert*] requirement is to ensure the reliability and relevancy of expert testimony. It is to make certain that an expert, whether basing testimony upon professional studies or *personal experience, employs in the courtroom the same level of intellectual rigor that characterizes the practice of an expert in the relevant field.* [emphasis added] (2, p. 1176)

In a concurring opinion that is important to the concerns of this chapter, Justice Scalia (joined by Justices O'Connor and Thomas) emphasized that the trial court's decision to admit or exclude an expert's testimony *is* reviewable for reasonableness:

> I think it is worth adding that it is not discretion to perform the function inadequately. Rather, it is discretion to choose among *reasonable* means of excluding expertise that is *fausse* [false] and science that is junky. Though, as the court makes clear today, the *Daubert* factors are not holy writ, in a particular case the failure to apply one or another of them may be unreasonable, and hence an abuse of discretion. [emphasis in original] (2, p. 1179)

Does *Daubert* Matter?

Although this chapter has taken the position that experts should be guided by the recent Supreme Court decisions in crafting their testimony, a recent special issue of the journal *Psychology, Public Policy, and Law* demurs from this view (10). The journal issue contains several commentaries and applications of *Daubert* to various forensic functions. The authors of the lead article note:

> Since *Daubert*, evidence has been excluded in isolated cases that would have been admitted pre-*Daubert*, but overall *Daubert* has not resulted in changes in the admissibility of behavioral and social science evidence. Conversely, behavioral and social science evidence that was admitted before *Daubert* has been admitted after . (11, pp. 4–5)

After this daunting conclusion, the authors go on to suggest that the *Daubert* decision (and, presumably, its progeny as well) may offer expert witnesses guidance on more than just the simple matter of courtroom admissibility. They state:

> *Daubert's* principle can be used to ask why it is that behavioral and social scientists consider it legitimate to do what it is that they do. Ironically, although judges can be criticized for not having sufficient expertise to judge the admissibility of behavioral and social scientific information, behavioral and social scientists can be criticized for not spending the time to analyze critically their own behavior to determine if they are engaging in acts or judgments that exceed their intrinsic expertise. (11, p. 14)

These last words constitute both a warning and a challenge to expert witnesses. The issues discussed here may stimulate experts to consider employing the suggestions noted below.

Recommendations

The foundation provided by the Supreme Court has encouraged the emergence of some concrete questions that may serve as self-tests for the expert:

1. Is the discipline advocated by the proffered witness a reliable one or one that is viewed clinically as the functional equivalent of phrenology? (2, p. 1175)
2. Is the methodology an accepted one and appropriately applied to the facts in the case? (Note the case example presented above as to

failure to consider collateral sources or to conduct a standard battery of psychological tests.)
3. In the psychology/psychiatry community is there a recognition of the legitimacy of one clinician's experience versus another's, for example, comparing a practitioner specializing in a narrow area to a generalist, or a senior to a junior clinician?

Comparably concrete suggestions have been proffered (see, for example, 10–13) as to how to address these questions:

1. First, expert opinion is strengthened by drawing upon recognized clinical entities, rather than on ad hoc novel entities that require departures from clinical traditions. This does not mean that innovation is not possible, only that it should be attempted with great care to avoid promiscuous creation of diagnostic entities to meet the needs of a particular case.
2. Literature review and the use of citations that are "on point" are extremely useful techniques for meeting the requirements of both a general acceptance standard and a scientific reliability standard. To perform their task adequately, forensic experts must be able to provide empirical/scientific/consensus bases for their opinions. Data that can fulfill these functions might be taken, for example, from open trials, clinical studies, task force reports on psychiatric testimony, official practice guidelines, consensus guidelines, and similar relevant sources.
3. The question of relevance does not flow from the professional literature but requires expert self-scrutiny beginning with the question, does psychiatry itself have anything to say about this case at all? If that question is answered in the affirmative, the expert must consider whether his or her particular expertise can assist the fact finder in understanding something relevant to the *legal* issue at hand. Such self-examination requires objectivity and freedom from narcissistic bias ("I have valuable opinions about everything").
4. Peer consultation, undertaken confidentially and anonymously, may be helpful in complex cases. However, it is unclear under what circumstances the fact of such consultation might be discoverable and unclear whether such discovery is necessarily an argument against doing it.

Conclusion

As noted, the effect of the recent Supreme Court cases described above is controversial: will they actually shape expert testimony in the new millennium? Given the authority and guidance offered by these decisions, however, particularly *Joiner* and *Kumho Tire,* the start of the present millennium is an excellent time to consider implementing their recommendations by building their standards into expert witness practice.

References

1. Huber P: Galileo's Revenge: Junk Science in the Courtroom. New York, Basic Books, 1991
2. Kumho Tire v Carmichael, 19 S Ct 1167 (1999)
3. Daubert v Merrell Dow Pharmaceuticals 509 US 579 (1993)
4. Gutheil TG, Stein MD: *Daubert*-based gatekeeping and psychiatric/psychological testimony in court: review and proposal. J Psychiatry Law 28:235–251, 2000
5. General Electric Co. v Joiner, 522 US 136, 118 S Ct 512 (1997)
6. Frye v United States, 54 App DC 46, 47, 293 F 1013, 1014 (1923)
7. Beech Aircraft Corp. v Rainey, 488 US 153, 169 (1988)
8. Feldman-Schorrig SP, McDonald JJ: The role of forensic psychiatry in the defense of sexual harassment cases. J Psychiatry Law 20:5–33, 1992
9. Pope KS, Butcher JN, Seelen J: The MMPI, MMPI-2 and MMPI-A in Court: A Practical Guide. Washington, DC, American Psychological Association, 1993
10. Shuman DW, Sales BD (eds): *Daubert's* meanings for the admissibility of behavioral and social science evidence. Psychology, Public Policy, and Law, special theme issue, 5:3–242, 1999
11. Shuman DW, Sales BD: The impact of *Daubert* and its progeny on the admissibility of behavioral and social science evidence. Psychology, Public Policy, and Law 5:3–15, 1999
12. Gutheil TG: The Psychiatrist as Expert Witness. Washington, DC, American Psychiatric Press, 1998
13. Gutheil TG, Bursztajn H: Avoiding *Ipse Dixit* mislabeling: post-Daubert formation of expert opinion. J Am Acad Psychiatry Law (in press)

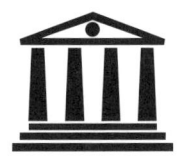

PART VI

Ethical Issues

11

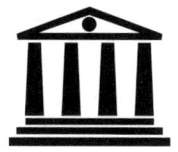

Some Ethical Dilemmas

> We [psychiatrists] may resist continuing post-graduate self-scrutiny, but it is particularly important in forensic practice because our foibles, biases, laxities or incautions are especially vulnerable to public attention.... If we fail to base our habitual performance on the dictum [of knowing our limitations], we risk being trapped in pitfalls of our own making.
>
> H.C. Modlin, in (1), p. 419

The ethics guidelines of the American Academy of Psychiatry and the Law (see Appendix 11–1) offer some general principles that may be of use to expert witnesses practicing their craft. An additional approach, with which the present authors concur, has been offered by Brodsky, who defines a four-level hierarchy of ethical duties for experts (2, p. 41). The first duty is to the truth of your findings, termed "the integrity of what you know" (2, p. 41). The second level of duty derives from your "codified obligations to the court" (2, p. 41)—

that is, to the rules established by the legal system.

The third level consists of "responsibility to the party being evaluated and to both sets of attorneys" (2, p. 41). This duty might include honesty about the limits of data, on direct or cross-examination. The final level of duty is "obligation to yourself and your profession" on the witness stand, including the duty to avoid compromise "of knowledge and findings" (2, p. 41).

Some common elements of the expert's ethical universe have been addressed elsewhere (3, 4) and alluded to in this book. This chapter addresses a few of the less common but more complex dilemmas an expert might encounter that defy clear resolution by the usual codes, presenting them in the form of vignettes. Each vignette is followed by some ethical questions that might arise from the dilemma. The reader should attempt his or her own answers to the questions before going on to the subsequent discussion.

Note that the analysis following each example does not pretend to constitute the definitive answer to the questions asked. Rather, it represents a reasonable approach that could be defended in court. The reader is invited to try making ethical arguments for both sides (i.e., pro and con) of each case vignette.

Case Examples, Questions, and Discussion

Example 1

An expert witness who holds a faculty position at a medical school is consulted by an attorney with regard to emotional injuries claimed by a plaintiff who is a faculty member at the parent university (but in a different department from the expert's). The plaintiff was a "whistleblower" concerning misuse of research funds and was subsequently fired. He became depressed as a result and is now bringing suit against the university for wrongful termination and related claims.

The expert is asked to address solely the emotional injuries, not questions of liability. However, to be retained by the plaintiff in this case is, in effect, to be on the side of litigation against his own parent university.

Questions

1. May the expert take the case? Should the expert take the case?
2. To what degree is there a conflict-of-interest issue? If you believe that one is present, what steps might mitigate it?
3. Is it relevant that the university would not want its own research

funds misused or its own faculty members punished inappropriately by termination?
4. Are whistle-blowers entitled to any special considerations, given the difficulty and value of their role?
5. Resnick has stated, "If a psychiatrist is on the clinical faculty of a medical school, he should inform the attorney of this fact before reviewing a malpractice suit against a teaching hospital associated with the school" (5, p. 3). In the context described above, Resnick's recommendation appears not to preclude participation in the case. Is this notification sufficient to mitigate any conflict-of-interest problems? Should it be?

Discussion

The most conservative position would be that whether or not there is a problem, the ethics of the situation are too cloudy to allow acceptance of the case; declining avoids even the appearance of a problem. This would follow the "unwritten rule," suggested by some scholars, of avoiding going against one's own university.

An alternative would be the "strict constructionist" position, permitting the expert to take the case on the grounds that universities are vast aggregates of departments and individuals, most of whom work in complete independence of each other. Therefore, as long as plaintiff and expert move in sufficiently different orbits, as they do in this case, there is no actual conflict.

A third model is the "therapeutic alliance" approach: the expert is opposing not his own university as such, but its venal, fraudulent, or even criminal elements. As a therapist supports the healthy side of the patient against the elements of illness in that very patient, the expert here would be siding with the righteous aspects of his university against its own improper actions and bad decision.

Yet another approach is the "high moral ground" argument. The whistle-blower is a precious commodity, deserving of support and protection against retaliation in any form. For this reason the expert should take the case regardless of the context.

The question also arises: why would the attorney, with a world of experts to choose from, select one from that very university? Was this an attempt somehow to bolster the case? Were other factors involved, such as previous work with that expert? Would those other factors outweigh the problems?

A valuable and possibly mitigating step for the expert might be discussion with medical school counsel, university counsel, or both. Permission might be given to take the case based on one of the above lines of argument.

Example 2

In a sexual misconduct case, a treating therapist is alleged to have had a sexual relationship with a patient who is herself an experienced therapist. A defense attorney consults the expert to work for the defense of the treater based on the following theory.

This jurisdiction operates under contributory negligence statutes, whereby any negligence by the plaintiff may vitiate the claim, leading to case dismissal. Therefore, if the therapist-plaintiff was aware the relationship was inappropriate but did not act to leave or terminate it, she has no claim. Evidence in the case indicates overwhelmingly that the therapist-plaintiff was fully aware of the wrongness of such a relationship. The expert, who strongly opposes sexual misconduct, considers whether she can take such a case on the offending treater's side.

Questions

1. What role does moral disapproval of a plaintiff, or, for that matter, a defendant, play in decisions faced by an expert witness? In other words, should the merit of a case or the appeal of the retaining attorney's client be paramount?
2. No expert can be compelled to take a case, yet everyone is constitutionally entitled to a defense. Is this a justification for taking the case? Should experts take cases when their feelings about an issue in the case may color their judgment?
3. According to the ethics guidelines of the American Academy of Psychiatry and the Law, forensic psychiatry involves application of "scientific and clinical expertise" to "legal issues in legal contexts" (Appendix 11–1, Preamble). Does this principle offer any guidance here?

Discussion

Again, an expert may always turn down a case because of discomfort with the issues or the parties involved. Should the expert decide to take the case, several principles may apply. First, everyone is, indeed, entitled to a defense. The moral struggle here may be the civil equivalent of testifying for the defense on grounds for insanity of a defendant who has committed a heinous criminal act.

A "strict constructionist" view might propose that the law says contributory negligence is grounds for dismissal. If the forensic evidence supports that finding, then there is no problem with so testifying. But given the recognized power of transference feelings, contributory negligence in this context may be a legal fiction rather than a legal principle.

Finally, when experts find themselves emotionally involved with a case, as they may be, consciously or unconsciously, at any time, the essential question—as with a case of any type—is whether any resulting bias can be managed. If the expert is so uncomfortable with the side of the case offering retention that impairment of forensic or clinical judgment is likely, the expert should decline the case.

Example 3

An expert uses "readers" or "screeners" to assist in the review of a case. The readers are either trainees or junior practitioners who are paid for their time by the expert. They wade through extensive case material, providing digests, summaries, or flagging of important data for the expert. The expert does the actual testifying.

Questions

1. Is this an ethical practice? Does it make a difference whether or not the senior expert himself does read the material at some point?
2. May, should, or must the retaining attorney be informed of the situation?
3. Assume that the retaining attorney has been informed and has no objection to this practice when informed; does this resolve the issue?
4. One scholar has informally suggested that this practice is acceptable and need not even be disclosed to the retaining attorney because attorneys use paralegals constantly for various tasks such as legal research and do not necessarily tell clients or experts about it. They may even bill as if they themselves had done the work billed for. Is this an acceptable defense?

Discussion

The practice described above is apparently not uncommon among experts but has not been openly discussed in forensic fora. The retaining attorney should probably be advised of the practice on the basis of "truth in billing" principles. This information allows the attorney to make a choice about the matter and perhaps decide to retain an expert who does all the work himself or herself. On the other hand, because screening may achieve greater efficiency, the attorney may prefer this approach as a way of minimizing costs, especially in cases with massive amounts of paperwork, such as toxic tort cases with large numbers of plaintiffs.

The practice of using screeners touches directly on the question of what services the expert is offering. Screening may allow the expert to rapidly zoom in on critical nuggets buried in the mass of data, but the expert's own knowledge, skill, and experience are not brought to bear in detecting subtle points that screeners may miss. This issue obviously turns on whether the expert ultimately does read all the material, perhaps later in the case review. If the expert has not read the database, the situation might be analogous to opining without examining an available litigant.

Finally, on cross-examination opposing attorneys may attempt to portray the expert's use of screeners as a pecuniary, business-oriented, mass-production procedure that precludes careful clinically based case review.

Example 4

In a malpractice case involving a patient's suicide on an inpatient unit of a community hospital, the plaintiff's expert, who serves as full-time faculty at a teaching institution, criticizes in detail the failings of the treaters and the hospital, holding both to an extremely high standard of practice. Not until deposition is it revealed that the expert last treated inpatients more than 30 years earlier.

Questions

1. Is this distance in time from actual inpatient work a bar to testimony? Is your answer different depending on whether the attorney knows this fact or not? Assuming the attorney does know but doesn't care, should the expert still care enough about this issue to pass the case on to a psychiatrist more intimately familiar with inpatient work?
2. Does working in a presumably cutting-edge teaching setting interfere with the ability to properly assess the standard of care in a community hospital? Is this a surmountable bias? Is it different from the posture of a typical hired gun who offers a "counsel of perfection" as though it were the standard?

Discussion

All experts who work in academic settings must beware of the "ivory tower" bias when dealing with nonacademic settings that may not necessarily fall below the standard of care, even though MRI (magnetic resonance imaging) scans are not instantly available and the more traditional medications may be used first. Experts must also avoid using "what would *I* do" as their standard, since they may adhere to higher standards of practice than those of the relevant benchmark, the "average reasonable practitioner."

The time span since the expert's last work in the exact field under consideration may go, as the attorneys say, to the weight of the testimony, rather than to whether it may be proffered. Whether that time span is truly disqualifying is a delicate question, requiring the expert's candid self-assessment, with advice from the retaining attorney. The matter may turn on the question of whether management of the suicidal inpatient has undergone profound changes in the intervening decades or whether the same fundamental principles may still apply.

References

1. Modlin HC: Forensic pitfalls. Bull Am Acad Psychiatry Law 17:415–419, 1989
2. Brodsky SL: The Expert Expert Witness: More Maxims and Guidelines for Testifying in Court. Washington, DC, American Psychological Association, 1999
3. Gutheil TG: The expert's ethical universe, in The Psychiatrist as Expert Witness. Washington, DC, American Psychiatric Press, 1998, pp 11–18
4. Gutheil TG: Ethics in forensic psychiatry, in Psychiatric Ethics, 3rd Edition. Edited by Bloch S, Chodoff P, Green S. Oxford, Oxford University Press, 1999, pp 345–361
5. Resnick PJ: The psychiatrist in court, in Psychiatry, Vol 3. Edited by Cavenar JO. Philadelphia, PA, JB Lippincott, 1986, pp 1–10

Appendix 11–1

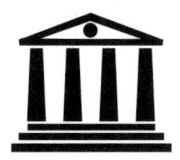

American Academy of Psychiatry and the Law Ethical Guidelines for the Practice of Forensic Psychiatry

I. Preamble

The American Academy of Psychiatry and the Law is dedicated to the highest standards of practice in forensic psychiatry. Recognizing the unique aspects of this practice which is at the interface of the professions of psychiatry and the law, the Academy presents these guidelines for the ethical practice of forensic psychiatry.

Reprinted from "American Academy of Psychiatry & the Law Ethical Guidelines for the Practice of Forensic Psychiatry," adopted May 1987; last revised 1995. See http://www.emory.edu/AAPL/ethics.htm. Accessed December 5, 2001. Reprinted with the permission of the American Academy of Psychiatry and the Law.

Commentary

Forensic Psychiatry is a subspecialty of psychiatry, a medical specialty. Membership in the American Psychiatric Association, or its equivalent, is a prerequisite for membership in the American Academy of Psychiatry and the Law. Hence, these guidelines supplement the Annotations Especially Applicable to Psychiatry of the American Psychiatric Association to the Principles of Medical Ethics of the American Medical Association.

The American Academy of Psychiatry and the Law endorses the Definition of Forensic Psychiatry adopted by the American Board of Forensic Psychiatry, Inc.

"Forensic Psychiatry is a subspecialty of psychiatry in which scientific and clinical expertise is applied to legal issues in legal contexts embracing civil, criminal, and correctional or legislative matters: forensic psychiatry should be practiced in accordance with guidelines and ethical principles enunciated by the profession of psychiatry." (Adopted May 20, 1985)

The forensic psychiatrist practices this subspecialty at the interface of two professions, each of which is concerned with human behavior and each of which has developed its own particular institutions, procedures, values, and vocabulary. As a consequence, the practice of forensic psychiatry entails inherent potentials for complications, conflicts, misunderstandings, and abuses.

In view of these concerns, the American Academy of Psychiatry and Law provides these guidelines for the ethical practice of forensic psychiatry.

II. Confidentiality

Respect for the individual's right of privacy and the maintenance of confidentiality are major concerns of the psychiatrist performing forensic evaluations. The psychiatrist maintains confidentiality to the extent possible given the legal context. Special attention is paid to any limitations on the usual precepts of medical confidentiality. An evaluation for forensic purposes begins with notice to the evaluee of any limitations on confidentiality. Information or reports derived from the forensic evaluation are subject to the rules of confidentiality as applied to the evaluation, and any disclosure is restricted accordingly.

Commentary

The forensic situation often presents significant problems in regard to confidentiality. The psychiatrist must be aware of and alert to those issues of privacy and confidentiality presented by the particular forensic situation. Notice should be given as to any limitations. For example, before beginning a forensic evaluation, psychiatrists should inform the evaluee that although they are psychiatrists, they are not the evaluee's "doctor." Psychiatrists should indicate for whom they are conducting the examination and what they will do with the information obtained as a result of the examination. There is a continuing obligation to be sensitive to the fact that although a warning has been given, there may be slippage and a treatment relationship may develop in the mind of the examinee.

Psychiatrists should take precautions to assure that none of the confidential information they receive falls into the hands of unauthorized persons.

Psychiatrists should clarify with a potentially retaining attorney whether an initial screening conversation prior to a formal agreement will interdict consultation with the opposing side if the psychiatrist decides not to accept the consultation.

In a treatment situation, whether in regard to an inpatient or to an outpatient in a parole, probation, or conditional release situation, psychiatrists should be clear about any limitations on the usual principles of confidentiality in the treatment relationship and ensure that these limitations are communicated to patients. Psychiatrists should be familiar with the institutional policies in regard to confidentiality. Where no policy exists, psychiatrists should clarify these matters with the institutional authorities and develop working guidelines to define their role.

III. Consent

The informed consent of the subject of a forensic evaluation is obtained when possible. Where consent is not required, notice is given to the evaluee of the nature of the evaluation. If the evaluee is not competent to give consent, substituted consent is obtained in accordance with the laws of the jurisdiction.

Commentary

Consent is one of the core values of the ethical practice of medicine and psychiatry. It reflects respect for the person, a fundamental principle in the practices of medicine, psychiatry, and forensic psychiatry. Obtaining informed consent is an expression of this respect.

It is important to appreciate that in particular situations, such as court-ordered evaluations for competency to stand trial or involuntary commitment, consent is not required. In such a case, the psychiatrist should so inform the subject and explain that the evaluation is legally required and that if the subject refuses to participate in the evaluation, this fact will be included in any report or testimony.

With regard to any person charged with criminal acts, ethical considerations preclude forensic evaluation prior to access to, or availability of legal counsel. The only exception is an examination for the purpose of rendering emergency medical care and treatment.

Consent to treatment in a jail or prison or other criminal justice setting must be differentiated from consent to evaluation. The psychiatrists providing treatment in these settings should be familiar with the jurisdiction's rules in regard to the patient's right to refuse treatment.

IV. Honesty and Striving for Objectivity

Forensic psychiatrists function as experts within the legal process. Although they may be retained by one party to a dispute in a civil matter or the prosecution or defense in a criminal matter, they adhere to the principle of honesty and they strive for objectivity. Their clinical evaluation and the application of the data obtained to the legal criteria are performed in the spirit of such honesty and efforts to attain objectivity. Their opinion reflects this honesty and efforts to attain objectivity.

Commentary

The adversarial nature of our Anglo-American legal process presents special hazards for the practicing forensic psychiatrist. Being retained by one side in a civil or criminal matter exposes the forensic psychiatrist to the potential for unintended bias and the danger of distortion of their opinion. It is the responsibility of forensic psychiatrists to minimize such hazards by carrying out their responsibilities in an honest manner striving to reach an objective opinion.

Practicing forensic psychiatrists enhance the honesty and objectivity of their work by basing their forensic opinions, forensic reports, and forensic testimony on all the data available to them. They communicate the honesty of their work, efforts to obtain objectivity, and soundness of their clinical opinion by distinguishing, to the extent possible, between verified and unverified information as well as among clinical "facts," "inferences," and "impressions."

While it is ethical to provide consultation to an adversary in a legal dispute as a testifying or reporting expert, honesty and striving for objectivity are required. The impression that psychiatrists in a forensic situation might distort their opinion in the service of the party which retained them is especially detrimental to the profession and must be assiduously avoided. Honesty, objectivity, and the adequacy of the clinical evaluation may be called into question when an expert opinion is offered without a personal evaluation. While there are authorities who would bar an expert opinion in regard to an individual who has not been personally examined, it is the position of the Academy that if, after earnest effort, it is not possible to conduct a personal examination, an opinion may be rendered on the basis of other information. However, under such circumstances, it is the responsibility of forensic psychiatrists to ensure that the statements of their opinions and any reports of testimony based on those opinions, clearly indicate that there was no personal examination and the opinions expressed are thereby limited.

In custody cases, honesty and striving for objectivity require that all parties be interviewed, if possible, before an opinion is rendered. When this is not possible, or if for any reason not done, this fact should be clearly indicated in the forensic psychiatrist's report and testimony. Where one parent has not been interviewed, even after deliberate effort, it may be inappropriate to comment on that parent's fitness as a parent. Any comments on that parent's fitness should be qualified and the data for the opinion be clearly indicated.

Contingency fees, because of the problems that these create in regard to honesty and efforts to attain objectivity, should not be accepted. On the other hand, retainer fees do not create problems in regard to honesty and efforts to attain objectivity and, therefore, may be accepted.

Treating psychiatrists should generally avoid agreeing to be an expert witness or to perform evaluations of their patients for legal purposes because a forensic evaluation usually requires that other people be interviewed and testimony may adversely affect the therapeutic relationship.

V. Qualifications

Expertise in the practice of forensic psychiatry is claimed only in areas of actual knowledge and skills, training, and experience.

Commentary

As regards expert opinions, reports, and testimony, the expert's qualifications should be presented accurately and precisely. As a correlate of the principle that expertise may be appropriately claimed only in areas of actual knowledge, skill, training, and experience, there are areas of special expertise, such as the evaluation of children or persons of foreign cultures, or prisoners, that may require special training and expertise.

VI. Procedures for Handling Complaints of Unethical Conduct

Complaints of unethical conduct against members of the Academy will be returned to the complainant with guidance as to where the complaint should be registered. Generally, they will be referred to the local district branch of the American Psychiatric Association (APA). If the member does not belong to the APA, the complainant will be referred to the state licensing board or to the psychiatric association in the appropriate country. If the APA, the American Academy of Child and Adolescent Psychiatry, or the psychiatric association of another country should expel or suspend a member, AAPL will also expel or suspend the member upon notification of such action, regardless of continuing membership status in other organizations. AAPL will not necessarily follow the APA or other organizations in other actions.

Commentary

It is the present policy of the American Academy of Psychiatry and Law not to adjudicate questions of unethical conduct against members or nonmembers.

General questions in regard to ethical practice in forensic psychiatry are welcomed by the Academy and should be submitted for consideration to the Committee on Ethics.

The Committee will issue opinions on general or hypothetical questions but will not issue an opinion on the ethical conduct of a specific forensic psychiatrist or about an actual case.

Should a specific complaint against a member be submitted to the Academy, it will be referred to the Chair of the Ethics Committee. The Chair will, in turn, generally direct the complainant to the ethics committee of the local district branch of the American Psychiatric Association, to the state licensing board, or to the psychiatric organization of other countries for foreign members.

The Academy, through its Committee on Ethics or in any other way suitable, will assist the local or national committee on ethics of the American Psychiatric Association, state licensing boards or ethics committees of psychiatric organizations in other countries in the adjudication of complaints of unethical conduct or the development of guidelines of ethical conduct as they relate to forensic psychiatric issues.

Epilogue

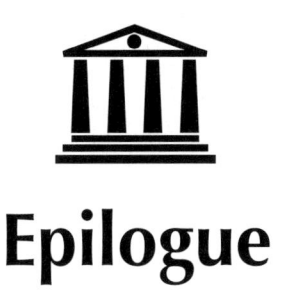

This text is designed to bring expert witnesses to a more advanced level of understanding of their field. Throughout the book we have attempted to illustrate—with empirical validation whenever possible—the issues and tensions that constitute an inescapable part of expert witness function. We have also tried to open to discussion a number of areas that—while thoroughly mined in informal conversations among experts—have not until now enjoyed the detailed disclosure and formal measurement in the literature that we attempt here.

In addition to opening new possibilities in forensic research, we hope to promote a dialogue with our attorney colleagues by pointing to areas of potential or actual conflict between attorney and expert in order to permit their clarification and resolution. The expansion of forensic psychiatric activity on all fronts makes this task of resolution even more urgent than in the past. We wish this book to further that goal.

The practice of forensic psychiatry is enormously challenging and interesting. Although it may hold many pitfalls for the unwary or forensically unsophisticated practitioner, forensic practice should be an enjoyable experience. We hope our book provides essential information that facilitates professional competence and satisfaction in the burgeoning specialty of forensic psychiatry.

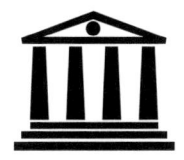

Suggested Readings

Babitsky S, Mangraviti JJ: How to Excel During Depositions: Techniques for Experts That Work. Falmouth, MA, SEAK, Inc., 1999

Babitsky S, Mangraviti JJ: How to Excel During Cross-Examination: Techniques for Experts That Work. Falmouth, MA, SEAK, Inc., 1999

Babitsky S, Mangraviti JJ, Todd CJ: The Comprehensive Forensic Services Manual: The Essential Resources for All Experts. Falmouth, MA, SEAK, Inc., 1999

A series of resources by two excellent teachers—attorneys who have worked extensively to present seminars and provide other resources for experts.

Brodsky SL: The Expert Expert Witness: More Maxims and Guidelines for Testifying in Court. Washington, DC, American Psychological Association, 1991

Brodsky SL: Testifying in Court: Guidelines and Maxims for Testifying in Court. Washington, DC, American Psychological Association, 1999

Two excellent books by a very senior forensic psychologist, both presented as brief discussions—often of topics not found elsewhere—summarized by a terse "maxim." Although the language level in Dr. Brodsky's examples is probably above the average jury's comprehension, these are excellent resources.

Feder HA: Succeeding as an Expert Witness: Increasing Your Impact and Income. Glenwood Springs, CO, Tageh Press, 1993

A wide-ranging, common-sense, detailed discussion of the work and life of an expert witness, by the late attorney and teacher.

Lifson L, Simon RI: The Mental Health Practitioner and the Law: A Comprehensive Handbook. Cambridge, MA, Harvard University Press, 1998

Aimed primarily at clinicians, this book has several chapters discussing the litigation context and courtroom work.

Lubert S: Expert Testimony: A Guide for Expert Witnesses and the Lawyers Who Examine Them. South Bend, IN, National Institute of Trial Advocacy, 1998

A highly recommended work addressed to experts and their retaining attorneys.

Malone DM, Hoffman PT: The Effective Deposition: Techniques and Strategies That Work, 2nd Edition. South Bend, IN, National Institute of Trial Advocacy, 1996

Malone DM, Zwier PJ: Expert rules: 100 (and More) Points You Need to Know About Expert Witnesses. South Bend, IN, National Institute of Trial Advocacy, 1999

Malone DM, Zwier PJ: Effective Expert Testimony. South Bend, IN, National Institute of Trial Advocacy, 2000

Three books by attorneys from the National Institute of Trial Advocacy, written from the viewpoint of the attorney as retainer of experts but valuable to forensic practitioners for that reason. Filled with tips and useful references, summaries of rules, etc.

Mulligan WG: Expert Witnesses: Direct and Cross-Examination. New York, Wiley, 1987

A comprehensive book by an attorney, with periodic update supplements.

Tsuhima WT, Anderson RW: Mastering Expert Testimony: A Courtroom Handbook for Mental Health Professionals. Mahwah, NJ, Erlbaum, 1996

A valuable book by two Hawaiian mental health professionals, presented in outline segments with copious referencing and crisp discussions.

Warren RA: The Effective Expert Witness: Proven Strategies for Successful Court Testimony. Lightfoot, VA, Gaynor Publishing, 1997

Not written from a psychiatric or medical perspective but contains various valuable points.

Index

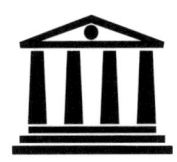

Page numbers printed in *boldface* type refer to tables and figures.

Abuse, sexual, disclosure of expert's, 106
Admissibility
 Daubert case, 114–117
 general acceptance test for, 115
 Joiner case, 117–119
 Kumho Tire case, 119–120
 self-tests for, 121–122
Advocacy
 avoidance of, 5
 boundary issues with, 24
Agreements, retainer. *See* Fee agreements
Ake v. Oklahoma, 101–102
Ambiguity, in forensics cases, 27
American Academy of Psychiatry and the Law
 ethics code, 109, 135–140
 informal surveys
  phantom experts, 68
 studies
  attorney-expert relations, 95–99
  attorney pressures, 58–63
  fee agreements, 37–39
American Arbitration Association, 34
American Medical Association, forensics classified by, 42

Approval, case example of expert's need for, 57–58
Assumed opinions, of attorneys, 49–50
 case example, 50
Attorney-expert relationships. *See also* Cross-examination
 countertransference in, 86–88
 empirical study of, 58–63
 ethics issues in, 63–65
 tension in, 47–58
  attorney-created, 49–55
  expert-related, 55–58
Attorney, opposing
 evidentiary limitations by, 8
 in examinations, 16–17
Attorney, retaining. *See* Retaining attorneys

Bar associations, complaints to, 63
Bias
 academic, case example, 132–133
 as countertransference, 81–82
 disclosure of expert's, 106
Board certification, 105
Bolstering, 7
Boundary negotiation, with attorneys, 24
Bribery, 55
Business arrangements, 4

145

Case examples
  assumed opinions, 50
  attorney complaints, 54
  clinical-forensic confusion, 15
  collateral sources, 8–9
  conflict of interest, 128–130
  countertransference, forensic, 82, 83
  countertransference, litigant, 88
  evidentiary limitations, 8
  expert's need for approval, 57–58
  fee concerns, 54
  inadequate assessment, 116
  inexperience, 57
  ivory tower bias, 132–133
  moral disapproval, 130–131
  phantom experts, 70, 73
  preoccupation with examinee, 84
  secondary PTSD, 85
  testimony without examination, 56
  use of screeners, 131–132
  zealousness, 58
Case files
  data withheld from, 59–60
  opinion offered prior to review of, 71
  time for reviewing, 25–26
Certification, board, 105
Child's Play (play), 88
A Civil Action (movie), 33
Clinician, role of v. expert, 6, 14–15
  case example, 15
Closing arguments, participation in, 29
Coercion, as influence, 61–63
Collateral sources, 8–9, 117
  case example, 8–9
Collections process, 34–35
Compensation. *See* Fees
Complaints
  to bar associations, 63
  of experts' unethical conduct, 140
  from retaining attorneys, case example, 54

Confidentiality, AAPL guidelines on, 136–137
Conflict of interest, case example, 128–130
Consent
  AAPL guidelines on, 137–138
  to examination, 15
  form, 21–22
Constraints, on examinations, 18–19
Consultants, experts as, 3–4
Consulting witness, role of, 4, 29
Contextual factors, exam in relation to, 17–18
Contingency fees, prohibition of, 35, 139
Contracts. *See* Fee agreements
Countertransference, clinical, 81
Countertransference, forensic
  attorney-centered, 86–88
  bias as, 81–82
  case examples, 82, 83
  contextual factors of, 88–89
  examinee-centered, 84–86
  expert's, 55–58
  litigant's, case example, 88
  positive effects of, 82
  remedies for, 89
Credentials. *See also* Disclosure
  AAPL guidelines on, 139–140
Critogenic factors, 17–18
Cross-examination
  attorney goals during, 94
  expert responses to, 95–99
  judicial rulings on, 99
"Crusher" depositions, 26–27
Custody cases, objectivity in, 139

Daubert v. Merrell Dow Pharmaceuticals, 114–117
  cited in *Kumho*, 120
  relevance of, 121
Defensiveness, with retaining attorney, 87–88
Depositions, planning for, 26–27

Index

Diagnostic and Statistical Manual of Mental Disorders, 7
Direct examinations, developing, 28
Disclosure
   about opposing experts, 101–111
      experts' views on, 103–108
      ethics issues in, 108–110
      limitations on, 102
Disclosure, expert, 69–70
Divorce
   cross-examination about, 95–96
   disclosure of expert's, 106
DSM (*Diagnostic and Statistical Manual of Mental Disorders*), 7

Empathy
   misuse of, 14
   as problematic, 85–86
Empirical studies
   AAPL
      attorney-expert relationships, 58–63
      cross-examination, 95–99
      disclosure of personal information, 103–108
      fee agreements, 37–39
   lacking in early forensics, xiii
   purpose of, xiv
Ethics guidelines
   AAPL, 109, 135–140
   Brodsky's hierarchy, 127–128
Ethics issues. *See also* Phantom practices
   advocacy, 5
   in attorney-expert relationships, 47–48, 63–65
   complaints regarding, 140
   confidentiality, 136–137
   conflict of interest, 128–130
   contingency fees, 35, 139
   disclosure. *See* Disclosure, ethics issues in
   experts' qualifications, 139–140
   informed consent, 137–138
   ivory tower bias, 132–133
   moral discomfort, 130–131
   nonpayment by attorneys, 35
   objectivity, 138–139
   testimony rehearsal, 27–28
   use of screeners, 131–132
   violation reporting, 76
Evidentiary limitations, case example, 8
Examinations, forensic
   consent to, 15
   constraints on, 18–19
   inadequate, 116–117
      case example of, 116
   nonclinical nature of, 14–15
   out-of-state
      fees for, 39
      license issues with, 42–43
   sites, 19
   teleconferenced, 43
   third parties in, 16–17
Expert disclosure, failure to share, 69–70
Expert-examinee relationship, nonclinical nature of, 14–15
Extortion, 55

Federal courts. *See individual cases*
Federal Rules of Civil Procedure, 118–119
Federal Rules of Evidence, 99, 115, 118–119
Fee agreements
   attorney modification of, 53
   empirical study of, 37–39
   guidelines for, 41–43
   suspicious language in, 49
   use of, 36–39
Fees
   case example of concern over, 54
   collection of, 33–35
   conflicts over, 51–52
   contingency, 35, 139
   sources of, 33
   ultimate responsibility for, 52

Fellowships, in forensic psychiatry, xiii
Filing deadlines, importance of, 72–73
Forensic psychiatry
  AMA classification of, 42
  defined by American Board of Forensic Psychiatry, 136
Freud, Sigmund, 23–24
Frye v. United States, 115

Gatekeeping
  implementation of, 119
  by lower courts, 114
General acceptance tests, for admissibility, 115
General Electric Co. v. Joiner, 117–119

Hate groups, membership in, 107
Hired guns, 56, 71

Income. *See also* Fees
  cross-examination about, 96–97
  sources of, 33
Inexperience, case example of expert's, 57
Information, selective withholding of, 50–51, 59–60
Injurious factors, of litigation, 17–18
Insurance, misinformation about, 52

Kumho Tire case, 114, 119–120

Litigation
  countertransference in, 88–89
  injurious factors of, 17–18

Malingering, 7, 15–16
Medical certainty, as testimonial standard, 5
Medicine, forensics deemed, 42–43
Money. *See also* Fees
  attitudes toward, 31–32
  conflicts over, 51–52
  countertransference reaction and, 86–87
Moral disapproval, case example, 130–131

Nontestifying witness, role of, 4, 29

Objectivity
  AAPL guidelines on, 138–139
  in ethics guidelines, 110
  tension from, 6
Opening statements, participation in, 29
Opinions
  in absentia. *See* Phantom practices
  assumed, of attorneys, 49–50
  persuasive statement of, 5
  prior to data review, 71
Opposing counsel
  evidentiary limitations by, 8
  in examinations, 16–17
Out-of-state work
  fees for, 39
  license issues with, 42–43
Outcomes, undue concern with, 86
Overidentification, with retaining attorney, 87
Overimmersion, in examinee's world view, 85–86

Parallels, between forensic cases, 73–74
Parsimony, 51–52
Partisan seduction, 60–61
Performance, testimony as, 6
Personal questions
  expert responses to, 95–99
  judicial rulings on, 99
Phantom practices, 67–77
  case examples, 70, 73
  defending, 73–74
  defined, 68
  legality of, 74–75
  motives for, 72–73
  strategies to combat, 75–77

Index

types of, 68–71
"Poker" depositions, 26
Posttraumatic stress disorder, secondary, 84–85
case example, 85
Preoccupation, with examinee, case example, 84
Privacy
AAPL guidelines on, 136–137
in examinations, 16–17
Program in Psychiatry and the Law studies
attorney pressures, 58–63
cross-examination, 95–99
disclosure, 103–108
fee agreements, 37–39
Protective orders, against personal questions, 99
Psychodynamic conflicts, over money, 51–52
Psychological testing, reliability of, 117

Qualifications, AAPL guidelines on, 139–140

Rates, 41–42. *See also* Fees
Recordings, of examinations, 16–17
Referrals, issues surrounding, 64–65
Reimbursement. *See* Fees
Reliability, scientific
establishing, 115–116
of psychological testing, 117
Religion, cross-examination about, 98
Retainers, 42. *See also* Fees
Retaining attorneys
bias toward, 65–66
bribery by, 55
business arrangements with, 4
complaints from, case example, 54
defensiveness with, 87–88
initial encounter with, 24
insufficient data provided by, 50–51

overidentification with, 87
payment problems with, 33–35
tension with, 47–48
and testimony preparation, 27

Schedules, negotiating, 25–26
Scientific reliability, 115–116, 117
Screening, ethics of performing, 131–132
case example, 131–132
of experts by attorneys, 50
Seductive power
of attorney, 60–61
of expert, 14–15
Sexual abuse, disclosure of expert's, 106
Sexual orientation
cross-examination about, 97–98
disclosure of expert's, 106
Sites, examination, 19
Skepticism, forensic, 15–16
Social context, tension from, 7
Studies, empirical
AAPL
attorney-expert relations, 58–63
cross-examination, 95–99
disclosure of personal information, 103–108
fee agreements, 37–39
lacking in early forensics, xiii
purpose of, xiv
Substance abuse
cross-examination about, 96, 97
disclosure of expert's, 106–107
Supreme Court. *See individual cases*
Surveys
AAPL, on phantom experts, 68

Teacher, expert as, 4–5
Telemedicine, 43
Testifying witness, role of, 4
Testimony
admissibility of. *See* Admissibility
limited by opposing counsel, 8

Testimony *(continued0*
　as performance, 6
　preparing, 27–28
　without examination, case
　　example, 56
Third parties, in examinations, 16–17
Threats, as influence, 61–63
Time, for case review, 25–26

Validation, expert's need for, 57–58
Venality, 56, 71

Whistle blowers, 129
Wills, cross-examination about, 97

Zealousness, case example of
　expert's, 58